the essentials in
hemodialysis

THE TARDIEU SERIES

the essentials in hemodialysis

Paul JUNGERS, M.D.

Associate Professor of Nephrology
Faculty of Medicine Necker-Enfants Malades
Necker Hospital
Paris

Johanna ZINGRAFF, M.D.

Chargée de Recherches
INSERM U 25
Necker Hospital
Paris

Nguyen K. MAN, M.D.

Maître de Recherches
INSERM U 25
Necker Hospital
Paris

Tilman DRUEKE, M.D.

Assistant Professor
Faculty of Medicine Necker
Necker Hospital
Paris

Bernard TARDIEU

Medical Illustrator

FOREWORD by George E. Schreiner, M.D.

Professor of Medicine
Director, Nephrology Division
Georgetown University School of Medicine, Washington, D.C.
President-elect, International Society of Nephrology
Editor, Transactions American Society
for Artificial Internal Organs, Inc.

1978
MARTINUS NIJHOFF MEDICAL DIVISION — THE HAGUE
— LONDON — BOSTON

WILLIAM MADISON RANDALL LIBRARY UNC AT WILMINGTON

© TARDIEU 1978
All rights reserved, including the right to translate or to reproduce this book or parts thereof in any form.
MARTINUS NIJHOFF MEDICAL DIVISION, 160 Old Derby Street, Hingham, MA 02043, U.S.
ISBN 90.247.21.03.2

FOREWORD

At the end of 1976 there were 34,215 people with end-stage renal disease alive on dialysis and transplantation within the registry centers of the European Dialysis and Transplant Association (14:4, 1977). From July, 1973, when the American Government began to fund dialysis, the estimated number of dialysis patients in the United States has risen from 5,000 plus to over 35,000. If we add other regions, such as Canada, Australasia and Latin America, it is safe to say that as this is written, over 100,000 people are living on dialysis.

The U.S. Social Security System, Veterans Administration, Medicaid and State Agencies are now paying out over one billion dollars annually to support patients on dialysis in the U.S.A. Cobe, Redy, Travenol, Dow Cordis, Drake Willock, Gambro, Asahi, Erica and a host of other company names have become household words in many households throughout the world.

I cite these factors not out of a pretense at precision or a passion for phenomenology, but simply to indicate that dialysis has become lore than this century's therapeutic miracle. (Perhaps the first treatable fatal chronic, terminal, medical disease !). It has also become big business ! As such, it has perhaps become too important to be left solely in the hands of medical specialists, such as nephrologists.

Accepting that thesis, how is one to disseminate deeply rooted bioengineering research, applied physiology, clinical investigation, organizational medicine and all the other components which have become the ingredients of a successful dialysis program ? Outside of the rather small circle of involved nephrologists are concentrically enlarging groups of other medical specialists, general physicians, house staff physicians, medical students, nurses, technicians, public health doctors, industry representatives and self-care dialysis patients who themselves must develop considerable technical knowledge and skills to survive their own care.

One way of beginning that educational venture is to have a reference manual giving both technical information and a how to do it approach in solving the problems in organizing and conducting dialysis.

This book is such a manual. It is a well organized effort from a very experienced dialysis group at the Necker Hospital in Paris under the leadership of Professor Jean Hamburger. The Topics are well organized in a highly logical manner beginning with the indications for dialysis, uremia, principles for hemodialysis, a definition of terms and an accurate description of dialysis equipment. Membrane, water, vascular access and patient problems are concisely covered. The adequacy of dialysis performance and the myriad problems with and complications seen in dialysis patients are discussed with frankness, thoroughness and sensitivity. Human and organizational considerations are not neglected.

This is a good book, timely and needed. Its fine translation into English should reach and enrich a large readership. When nephrologists are asked the oft recurring question, « What can I read ? », this is a manual to which they can point with pride.

> *George E. Schreiner, M.D.*
> *Professor of Medicine*
> *Director, Nephrology Division*
> *Georgetown University School of Medicine Washington, D.C.*
> *President-elect, International Society of Nephrology*
> *Editor, TRANSACTIONS, American Society*
>   *for Artificial Internal Organs, Inc.*

TABLE OF CONTENTS

FOREWORD	5
PREFACE	9

I - INDICATIONS FOR REGULAR DIALYSIS TREATMENT 11
1.1. Criteria for initiating chronic hemodialysis 11
1.2. Kidney diseases which lead to chronic hemodialysis 11
1.3. Evaluating hemodialysis requirements 12

**II - THE CONSEQUENCES OF LOSS OF RENAL FUNCTION:
THE MECHANISMS OF « UREMIC TOXICITY »** 13
2.1. The results of loss of excretory function 13
2.2. Consequences of the decreased water and electrolyte excretion 16
2.3. The results of the loss of endocrine and metabolic functions 17

III - BASIC PRINCIPLES OF HEMODIALYSIS 19
3.1. The Dialyzer 19
3.2. Diffusion (or conduction) transfer 20
3.3. Ultrafiltration (or convection) transfer 21
3.4. Flow rates and pressure 24
3.5. Evaluating dialyzer performance 25

IV - HEMODIALYSIS EQUIPEMENT 28
4.1. Dialyzers 28
4.2. Dialysate delivery systems and monitoring devices 29
4.3. The dialysate fluid 30
4.4. The special case of hemofiltration 35
4.5. Dialyzer performance 35

V - VASCULAR ACCESS
5.1. The main types of vascular access 37
5.2. Complications involved in vascular access 37

VI - ORGANIZATION OF DIALYSIS TREATMENT 40
6.1. Modalities of chronic hemodialysis 40
6.2. Preparation for regular dialysis treatment 40
6.3. Individual protocol for treatment 41

**VII - PERFORMANCE AND FOLLOW-UP OF REGULAR
DIALYSIS TREATMENT** 48
7.1. Performance of the hemodialysis session 48
7.2. Incidents and accidents during the hemodialysis session 52
7.3. Clinical and biochemical control of the hemodialysis patient 60

VIII - CLINICAL PROBLEMS IN CHRONIC HEMODIALYSIS PATIENTS . 70
- 8.1. **Cardiovascular problems** 70
- 8.2. **Hematological problems** 73
- 8.3. **Neurologic complications** 74
- 8.4. **Disorders of phospho-calcic metabolism** 78
- 8.5. **Infectious problems** 81
- 8.6. **Metabolic and endocrine problems** 82
- 8.7. **Gastrointestinal problems** 84
- 8.8. **Surgery in the dialysis patient** 85
- 8.9. **Dialysis in high-risk patients** 85
- 8.10. **Dialysis in the child** 86

IX - LIVING WITH HEMODIALYSIS 87
- 9.1. **Overall results of chronic hemodialysis** 87
- 9.2. **Diet of the hemodialyzed patient** 87
- 9.3. **The quality of life of the dialyzed patient** 88
- 9.4. **Social and professional rehabilitation** 88
- 9.5. **Economic consequences of the treatment** 89

SUBJECT INDEX 90

TABLE OF PLATES 96

REFERENCES 97

THE ESSENTIALS IN HEMODIALYSIS

PREFACE

Hemodialysis is an exchange that takes place between a patient's blood and an electrolyte solution similar to normal blood, across semipermeable membrane. This exchange removes wastes from the patient's blood an brings electrolyte balance to near normal. When hemodialysis is repeated regularly several times a week (whence the term « regular dialysis treatment » or « maintenance hemodialysis ») it theoretically can provide unlimited survival to patients whose own kidneys no longer function.

Hemodialysis treatment was initially restricted to patients with short-term acute renal failure, for at each session catheters had to be surgically implanted into an artery and a vein. Thus, the number of sessions per patient was limited. In 1960, B.H. Scribner and W.E. Quinton succeeded in short-circuiting the arterial blood into a vein with cannulae which could be left in place for repeated dialysis sessions.

This advance at first was greeted with scepticism, but its long-term success, as wall as that of renal transplantation which is contemporary, created a real revolution in the treatment of end-stage renal failure. Chronic hemodialysis was at first confined to a small number of patients, but since then it has grown to the point where more than 60,000 uremic patients throughout the world are surviving on chronic hemodialysis.

This relatively short period was one of great technical strides which cut the length of dialysis time required while making dialysis safer and more efficacious. In its wake followed extensive research into the mechanisms of the clinical disorders of renal insufficiency and this too has brought great progress in the treatment of renal insufficiency at each stage.

1 - INDICATIONS FOR REGULAR DIALYSIS TREATMENT

In the following chapters, regular dialysis treatment (RDT) will also be referred to as « chronic hemodialysis ».

1.1. Criteria for initiating chronic hemodialysis.

The aim of chronic hemodialysis is to allow the survival of patients whose chronic renal insufficiency has reached end-stage. This stage is usually defined by a reduction in glomerular filtration rate to under 5 ml/min [1,2]. This corresponds to less than 5 % of normal nephron function. In end-stage failure, glomerular filtration can be estimated from the mean of urea und creatinine clearance in the 24 hour urine collection. In practice, it is usually reflected, in the adult patient, by a blood creatinine level of 13 to 15 mg/100 ml.

In the early days of chronic hemodialysis, dialysis facilities were limited, and priorities for acceptance of patients had to be established. Those accepted were usually young adults who were heads of families, had no severe extrarenal complications and were considered to be capable of good rehabilitation with the aid of chronic hemodialysis [3]. Today, in most developed countries, enough facilities exist so that no selection has to be made based on type of kidney disease, age, sex, or economic status of patients [4].

However, some medical contra-indications to chronic hemodialysis do remain. They are due to the limitations inherent to the technique. Thus chronic hemodialysis is not usually recommended for patients who are physiologically aged or who have an irreversible decline in general physical state, severe impairment of mental faculties, severe and incurable psychic disorders, marked coronory insufficiency, or advanced malignancies. On the other hand, a greater freedom of choice is possible with aged patients or those with a systemic disease. When a good physical status has been retained and no major extrarenal complications exist, there is no fundamental contra-indication to chronic hemodialysis, but it should be recalled that these cases will constitute « high risk » dialysis [4]. Thus, in each patient, the decision for or against chronic hemodialysis should be made based on the predictable risks involved in treatment against the quality of life which can be expected.

1.2. Kidney diseases which lead to chronic hemodialysis (pl. 1).

« Primary » kidney diseases, i.e. those involving only the kidneys or urinary system, are the most frequent causes of renal destruction, accounting for more than 90 % of patients treated by chronic hemodialysis. Glomerulonephritis represents about 40 % of these primary diseases ; its incidence is significantly higher in males than in females, suggesting either a higher incidence or a more rapid evolution of glomerular diseases in males. Females, however, have a higher incidence of chronic pyelonephritis [4,6].

The incidence of the different types of kidney diseases observed in chronic dialysis patients admitted to the program of Necker Hospital and associated centers [4] is similar to the overall percentages reported for France [5], Europe [6] or the U.S.A. [7]. It may be noted that the percentage of patients with renal failure secondary to systemic diseases has grown from about 1 % ten years ago [8], to more than 10 % for patients admitted to RDT during 1976 [6].

In the last 15 years a clear-cut increase has been seen in the mean age of patients admitted to chronic hemodialysis treatment (Fig. 1). Between 1964 and 1971, the number of patients over 50 years in our series was below 15 % ; then, between 1972 and 1975 these patients made up 33 % of dialysis patients, and today their number exceeds 40 % of our new patients [4]. A similar development has been observed all over the world. Thus, the hemodialysis patient population is growing older and this longevity is furthermore increased by hemodialysis treatment itself. Related to this greater age and longevity is a modification in at least some of the types of complications observed among dialysis patients.

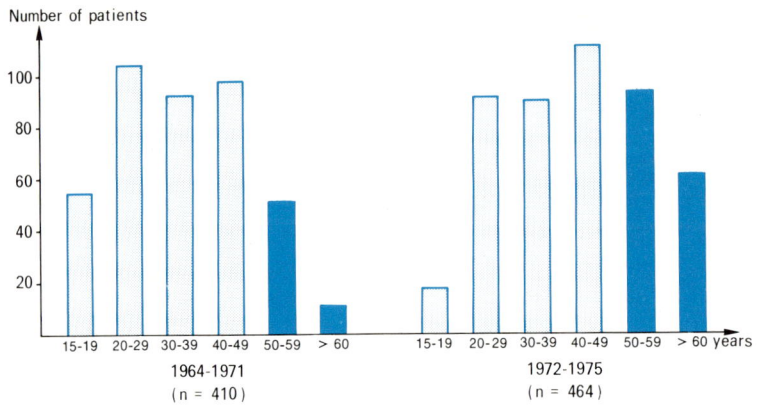

Fig. 1 - Age of patients at initiation of dialysis. (Necker hospital and associated centers).

1.3. Evaluating hemodialysis requirements

Requirements for hemodialysis are based on the number of new patients who each year reach end-stage renal failure. It is estimated to be 50 to 60 new patients per year per million inhabitants, when no limitations pertaining to age are considered [9].

Given the long survival of patients on maintenance hemodialysis, the number of posts required is large. It can be reduced only by successful renal transplantation. Thus, renal transplantation should be considered for every hemodialysis patient under 50 years of age. After 50, only exceptional cases should receive transplants, because of markeldly diminished tolerance to immunosuppressive treatment [1].

II — THE CONSEQUENCES OF LOSS OF RENAL FUNCTION :

THE MECHANISMS OF « UREMIC TOXICITY »

Normal kidneys perform three basic functions : excretion of the waste products of nitrogen metabolism ; regulation of water and electrolyte balance and, last but not least, endocrine and metabolic functions whose importance was more recently understood.

Since chronic hemodialysis is a purely physical process, it can substitute, at least in part, for the loss of the first two functions. However, endocrine and metabolic functions are beyond the scope of dialysis, for they require the presence of a functioning renal parenchyma.

We will discuss below the results of partial or total loss of the renal function reflected by a residual glomerular filtration rate of less than 5 ml/min, that is in end-stage renal failure. As a matter of comparison, as far as waste products are concerned, hemodialysis produces a status similar to that of a patient with a glomerular filtration rate near 20 ml/min.

The successive stages in renal insufficiency, beginning with normal function and progressing to end-stage renal failure, are shown in plate 2.

2.1. The results of loss of excretory function

In a normal subject, all the metabolites resulting from nitrogen catabolism are eliminated by the kidneys. In renal insufficiency, these metabolites accumulate in the blood and the tissues, proportionally to the degree of loss of renal function. Their toxicity is responsible for many of the clinical and biochemical disorders seen in uremic patients. However, it is not yet possible to precisely incriminate one or several of the individual metabolites as being at the origin of the clinical disorders related to uremia [10].

2.1.1. Urea, creatinine and uric acid

Quantitatively, urea is the most important of the nitrogen metabolites. It diffuses freely through all the water compartments of the body ; its intracellular concentration is as high as that in the blood. The result is a considerable accumulation of urea within the body of a uremic patient. The total body urea pool can be estimated by multiplying blood urea concentration by total body water (approximately 60 % of body weight). Thus, in a given patient weighing 70 kg and having a blood urea concentration of 300 mg/100 ml, the accumulated total body urea is approximately 120 g. As long as blood urea concentration remains below 300-400 mg/100 ml, it has no toxic effect per se. At concentrations above this level, urea may induce digestive and neurological manifestations such as nausea, vomiting, diarrhea and drowsiness [11].

Creatinine and uric acid have no toxic effects at concentrations occurring in clinical practice [12]. However, uric acid accumulation can cause gout (« secondary gout »).

2.1.2. Other low molecular weight nitrogen metabolites

Many other metabolites of nitrogen catabolism have been identified in the plasma of uremic patients [10]. Only the main substances will be mentioned.

— *Guanidine compounds* derive from the urea cycle and are the second largest group of protein catabolites. Three of them have proven toxic effects :

- *Guanidinosuccinic acid* inhibits the activation of platelet factor 3 and platelet aggregation. It may be play a part in the bleeding tendency seen in advanced uremia [13].
- *Methylguanidine* has been shown experimentally to cause neurological and digestive disorders.
- *Guanidinoproprionic acid* in vitro depresses glucose-6-phosphate dehydrogenase activity of red blood cells, altering their resistance to oxidants. It may thus be involved in the increased autohemolysis seen in uremic patients.

— *Phenolic compounds* are thought to be implicated in uremic thrombopathy and to inhibit the activity of several brain enzymes. They exhibit a high affinity to plasma proteins and thus a poor diffusion through dialysis membranes despite their low molecular weight.

— *Aliphatic amines,* notably dimethyl and trimethylamine are considered to be neurotoxic.

— *Myoinositol,* which was recently identified, has been shown to be neurotoxic in vitro, but its in vivo effects are still controversial.

— *Ammonia* is produced from the urea of intestinal fluid by gut bacterial ureases. When blood urea is in excess of 300 mg/100 ml, increased concentration of ammonia close to the intestinal mucosa may be responsible for digestive disorders [14].

Most of the above-mentioned metabolites have a low molecular weight, below 500 daltons. They thus diffuse easily across dialysis membranes, with the exception of those which are highly bound to proteins, such as the phenols.

2.1.3. High molecular weight toxins : « middle molecules ».

The above toxins explain only a part of the disorders observed in chronic renal insufficiency. If these disorders resulted only from freely diffusable, low molecular weight toxins, they should be totally corrected by chronic hemodialysis. However, some complications, such as uremic polyneuritis, may persist or even occur in patients treated by chronic hemodialysis, even when removal of urea and other low molecular weight waste products appears sufficient, whereas polyneuritis is always improved following successful renal transplantation [15].

These facts have suggested the possible responsibility of higher molecular weight metabolites, which are less quickly eliminated across the usual dialysis membranes. From these observations was born the « middle molecule » hypothesis, fathered by Scribner and Babb [16]. They observed that while « inadequate » hemodialysis often leads to uremic polyneuritis, the latter is not seen in patients on chronic peritoneal dialysis, despite higher urea and creatinine blood levels. They also noted that the peritoneal membrane is much more permeable to middle molecules than is the Cuprophan® membrane. This is also true, to a lesser degree, for molecules as heavy as 5,000 daltons. Based on these observations, Scribner and Babb hypothesized that uremic polyneuritis may be due to toxins between 500 and 2,000 daltons, which they called « middle molecules ». Although the chemical nature of these substances has not yet been elucidated and even their existence is controversial, the hypothesis proved to be a potent stimulus for work on understanding the manifestations of uremic toxicity.

For theoretical reasons (which are discussed in detail later) it is thought that the removal of these solutes is less dependent on the rate of blood or dialysate flow, than on the surface area of the membrane used and the number of hours of dialysis. This concept was expressed by Babb and Scribner as the « square meter — hour » hypothesis [16]. Two clinical observations support this hypothesis. First, in dialyzed patents who have polyneuritis, intensifying dialysis by increasing the weekly dialysis duration or by increasing membrane surface area results in clinical improvement. Second, the use of membranes with high permeability for middle molecules, such as polyacrylonitrile, improves an existing polyneuritis or precludes its development, without increasing dialysis time [17].

Subsequently, Bergström's team using high performance gel chromatography demonstrated electively high peaks corresponding to about 1,500 dalton molecules in the plasma of dialysis patients who had a poor general status, malnutrition, or episodes of pericarditis or infection [18]. At Necker Hospital, chromatographic analysis of the plasma ultrafiltrate of uremic patients showed a markedly pronounced peak only in those suffering from polyneuritis. This peak has been called fraction b4 and corresponds to a molecular weight of 1,300 to 1,500 daltons [19]. It rapidly disappears after the first few dialysis sessions (Fig. 2). A similar peak has also been found in the urine of healthy subjects, but not in their plasma. Studies are in progress to attempt to identify the neurotoxic substance(s) which compose this plasma fraction.

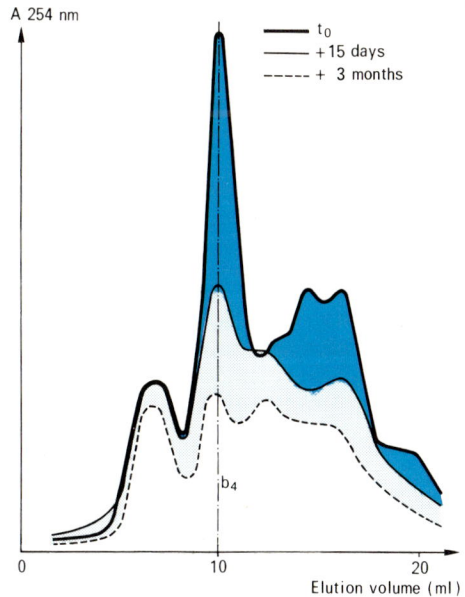

Fig. 2 - Plasma chromatography on Sephadex DEAE A25 from a dialysed patient with severe polyneuropathy. Decrease of peak « b4 » following intensive hemodialysis.

2.1.4. Other mechanisms involved in uremic toxicity

Two other mechanisms, which are not a direct result of the retention of toxic metabolites, are involved in certain uremic manifestations.

— The first is related to *hormonal changes* observed in uremia, such as elevated plasma levels of parathyroid hormone or glucagon, mainly due to defective hormone catabolism in the diseased kidneys (plate 3). This increase leads to important metabolic disturbances. According to N.S. Bricker's « trade-off hypothesis », it is the « price to pay » for attempting to maintain electrolyte balance [20]. The disadvantages of an increased level of circulating hormones, particularly parathyroid hormone, far outweigh its advantages.

— The second is the effect of urea retention on the stimulation of some *intermediary enzymes* of nitrogen metabolism. There is an increase in guanidine derivatives, as well as urea synthesis by the liver, and probably also of middle molecules ; on the other hand, the synthesis of muscular proteins is decreased. Thus, the alterations in nitrogen metabolism in uremia result in increased production of toxic nitrogen waste products and an undesirable reduction in the muscular mass [21].

2.2. Consequences of the decreased water and electrolyte excretion.

Up to a very advanced stage of renal insufficiency, residual nephrons exhibit a remarkable ability to regulate the excretion of electrolytes and water, thus maintaining the electrolyte and water balance of the organism [22]. However, when the number of functioning nephrons falls to below 5 % of normal, adaptation is no longer possible. In that case, neither waste removal nor water and electrolyte balance can be correctly maintained. Clinical and biochemical signs of uncompensated uremia appear, and the replacement of kidney functions by chronic hemodialysis becomes necessary (pl. 2).

When a uremic patient begins maintenance hemodialysis, diuresis usually decreases because the osmotic load, due to urea, is reduced. Urinary output becomes generally less than 1,000 ml/day. It may even be reduced to zero.

> **It results that in dialysis patients, electrolyte and water balance becomes entirely or almost entirely dependent on hemodialysis.**

2.2.1. **Water :** It accumulates between dialyses and is eliminated only by ultrafiltration during the following dialysis session. Any excessive fluid intake leads to an immediate expansion of body fluid volume. When taking into account insensible respiratory losses, a satisfactory fluid volume balance is usually achieved by ingestion of 500-700 ml of water above the amount of residual diuresis. Thus, in a hemodialysis patient having a mean daily urinary output of 500 ml, fluid intake would be approximately 1,000-1,200 ml per day.

2.2.2. **Sodium :** The problem of sodium excretion is similar to that of water. Sodium concentration in residual diuresis is most often about 50 mEq/l. Most of the sodium ingested between dialyses has to be removed by ultrafiltration during the following dialysis session.

2.2.3. **Potassium :** Potassium contained in food (or which can be produced by an excessive endogenous catabolism) leads to a rapid increase in its extracellular concentration and can result in lifethreatening hyperkalemia. Urinary excretion is very low. Thus, the accumulated potassium has to be removed during dialysis but often has also to be decreased by the ingestion of exchange resins between dialysis sessions.

2.2.4. **Bicarbonates :** The 60 to 100 milliequivalents of H^+ ions daily originating from intermediate metabolism are buffered by plasma bicarbonates Regeneration of plasma bicarbonate is provided by the acetate ions in the dialysis fluid, which are converted into bicarbonate by the liver and other tissues.

> **Thus, it is clear that water, sodium and potassium intake should be appropriately restricted between dialysis sessions.**

2.3. The results of the loss of endocrine and metabolic functions.

The main endocrine functions [23] which are reduced or lost at end-stage renal failure as shown on plate 3, are:

— production or activation of *erythropoietin,* the renal hormone which stimulates medullary red blood cell production. Because of strikingly decreased plasma erythropoietin levels, bilaterally nephrectomized patients have particularly severe anemia;

— hydroxylation of 25 OH *vitamine* D_3 to the active metabolite, 1, 25 $(OH)_2$ vitamine D_3, which stimulates intestinal absorption of calcium and phosphorus and is needed for skeletal mineralization [24];

— *renin-angiotensin system,* which is variably impaired. In some cases (particularly in patients with vascular or glomerular kidney diseases), excessive renin secretion can lead to persistent arterial hypertension. In others (especially anephric patients), the lack of renin secretion often induces a tendency to permanent hypotension.

The decrease or loss of metabolic functions of the kidney is responsible for impaired *inactivation of peptide hormones* such as insulin, glucagon, calcitonin, and parathyroid hormone, and contributes to the increased potentially toxic plasma levels of these hormones.

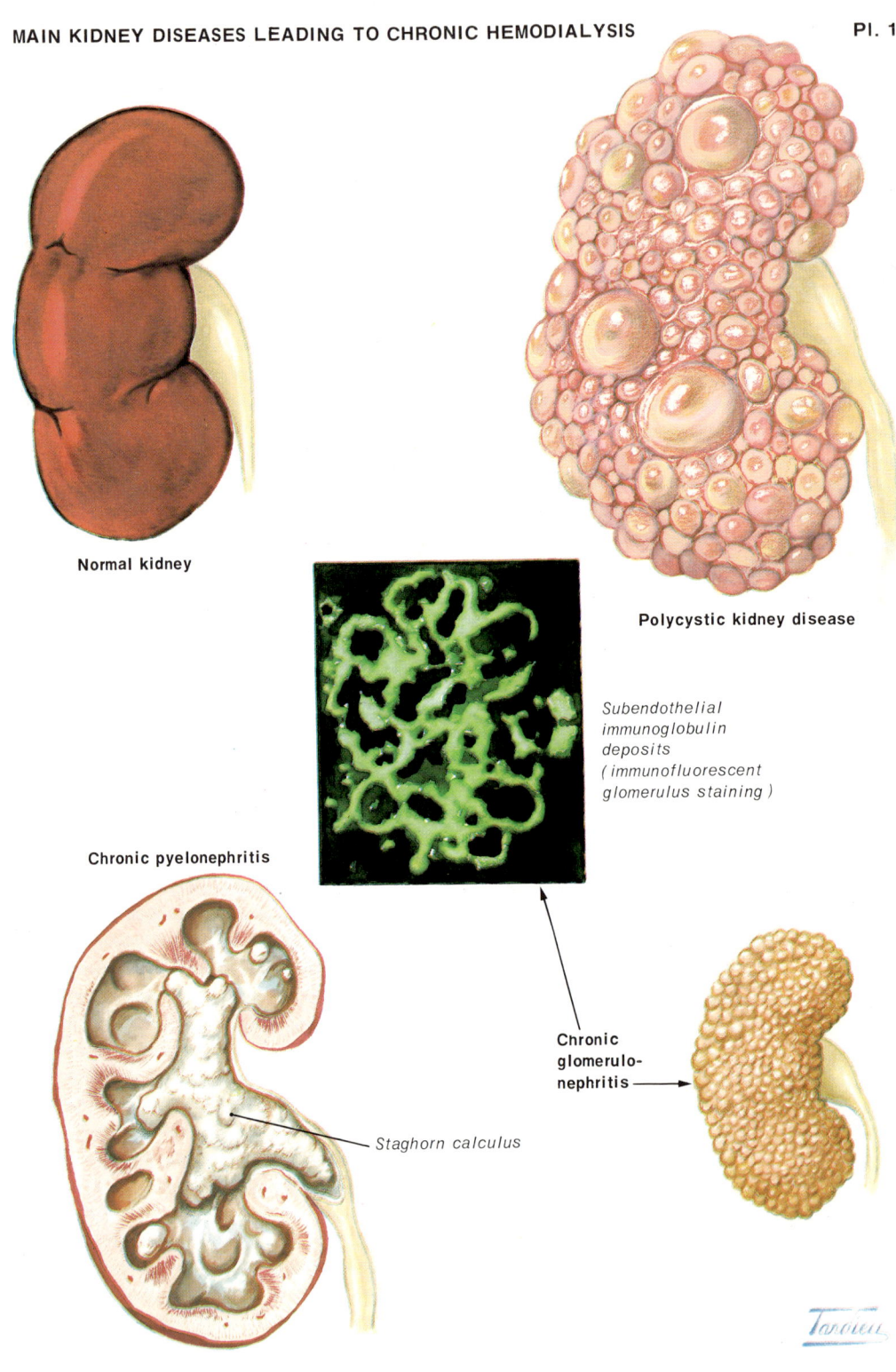

III — BASIC PRINCIPLES OF HEMODIALYSIS

Chronic hemodialysis replaces the excretory functions and the water and electrolyte homeostasis functions performed by the healthy kidney. This is achieved by a discontinuous exchange of water and solutes across a semipermeable membrane, separating the patient's blood from the dialysate fluid, whose composition is close to that of normal extracellular fluid. A hydrostatic pressure gradient may be created between the blood and the dialysate to remove by ultrafiltration the excess water and salt accumulated between dialysis sessions [25].

3.1. The Dialyzer

The dialyzer is the device where the exchange between the blood and the dialysis fluid takes place. Basically, it is made of a semipermeable membrane separating two compartments, one in which flows the patients' blood and the other the dialysis fluid (Fig. 3). The symbols QB and QD respectively designate the flow rates of the blood and the dialysis fluid; CB and CD stand for the concentration of each of them; the indices i and o show inflow into or outflow from the dialyzer.

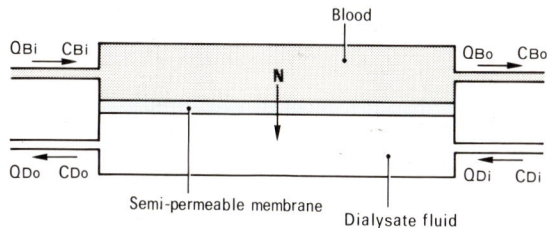

Fig. 3 - Schematic representation of a dialyzer.

The amount of solute transfer is calculated according to the laws of mass transfer across a semipermeable membrane [26] *Mass solute transfer* is the quantity of a solute transferred from the blood toward the dialysis fluid (or vice versa) per unit of time. The direction of the transfer is determined by the respective concentrations of the solute in the blood and the dialysis fluid (pl. 4), as well as by the pressure exerted on either side of the membrane.

The amount of solute removed from the blood in a given period of time (N) is the difference between the concentration of that solute entering the dialyzer ($C_{Bi} \times Q_{Bi}$) and that found at the outflow ($C_{Bo} \times Q_{Bo}$) [27], or:

$$N = (C_{Bi} \times Q_{Bi}) - (C_{Bo} \times Q_{Bo})$$

The amount of solute removed from the blood is, of course, equal to that found in the dialysis fluid at the same time, or:

$$N = (Q_{Do} \times C_{Do}) - (Q_{Di} \times C_{Di})$$

These formulae are used to evaluate the performance of dialyzers, which will be discussed below.

Mass transfer across semi-permeable membranes involves two basic mechanisms: diffusion (or conduction transfer) and ultrafiltration (or convection transfer).

3.2. Diffusion (or conduction) transfer

> **Diffusion transfer is a passive transfer of solutes across a membrane, in the absence of net solvent transfer.**

The amount of solute crossing a membrane by diffusion (Nd) depends on three factors [28]:

$$Nd = Ko \times A \times \overline{\Delta CM}$$

3.2.1. The mean concentration gradient of the solute on either side of the membrane ($\overline{\Delta CM}$). For maximum transfer, it should be as high as possible. This is the case when a given solute is absent from the dialysis fluid, such as in single pass, counter-current flow dialysis.

3.2.2. The effective dialysis surface area (A) is the part of the membrane effectively available for diffusion. This area can be increased by designs which, for instance, reduce corners where blood does not circulate. It is also possible to use several dialyzers in parallel or dialyzers having membranes of larger surface. The limiting factor in each case is the volume of extracorporeal blood required. The volume of extracorporeal circulation must not exceed that well tolerated by the patient, that is approximately 300 ml.

3.2.3. Total dialyzer permeability coefficient (Ko) determines mass transfer of a solute across the dialyzer. In order to move from the blood to the dialysis fluid, each molecule must diffuse first through the blood, then the dialysis membrane and finally the dialysis fluid. Each of these compartments opposes resistance to this transfer, symbolized as follows : RB, RM and RD (pl. 4). Overall or total resistance (Ro) is the sum of the individual resistances of all three compartment [29], or :

$$Ro = RB + RM + RD$$

Overall permeability coefficient (Ko) is the inverse of total resistance, or :

$$Ko = 1/Ro$$

To increase transfer by diffusion, the resistance of each compartment must be reduced as much as possible.

— RB can be lowered by reducing the active height of the blood channel. Initially as much as 400 microns in early plate dialyzers, new supporting structure designs have brought it to only 150 microns ; in hollow-fiber dialyzers it is now as little as 100 microns.

— RD can be reduced by increasing dialysate flow rate, which results in faster replacement of the fluid layers bordering the membrane. This flow rate reaches 0.5 to 1 liter per minute in plate or hollow-fiber dialyzers, and up to 30 liters per minute in coil dialyzers using a fluid recirculation system.

— RM for a given synthetic membrane can be reduced by decreasing its thickness, the limiting factor here being its physical resistance. The thickness of Cuprophan membranes has been reduced from about 30 to 10 microns. In addition, new synthetic membranes have been made, such as polyacrylonitrile and polycarbonate. Their permeability to all solutes is higher than that of Cuprophan, particularly to those with molecular weights above 1,000 daltons. This considerably reduces membrane resistance to middle molecules.

In conclusion, diffusion transfer varies considerably from one solute to another. The lower the molecular weight, the higher the rate of transfer. Moreover, the respective influence of RM, RB and RD in the overall dialyzer resistance to diffusion transfer varies according to solute molecular weight, and to the chemical nature of the membrane (pl. 5). Using Cuprophan® membranes, RM has a reduced part in the overall resistance to low molecular weight solutes such as urea or creatinine (Fig. 4a), where as it represents more than 50 percent of overall resistance for « middle » or high molecular weight solutes, such as vitamine B_{12} or inulin (Fig. 4b). Also, newer membranes such as polyacrylonitrile, polycarbonate or methylacrylate possess a much lower membrane resistance to middle or high molecular weight molecules than does Cuprophan®.

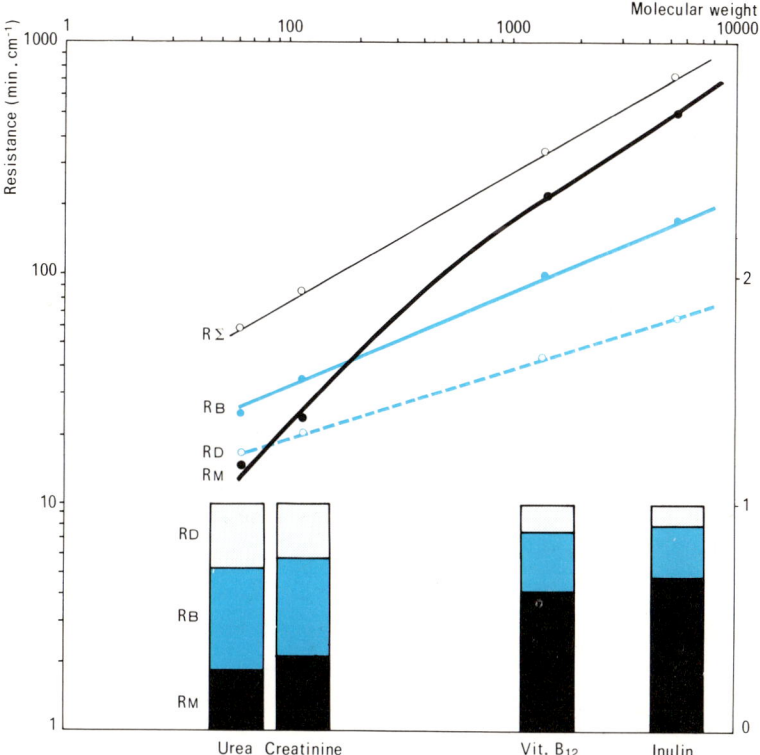

Fig. 4 - Growing part of RM amongst overall resistance to solute transfer, as solute molecular weight increases.

3.3. Ultrafiltration (or convection) transfer

Ultrafiltration is the simultaneous transfer of a solvent, with a part of the solutes it contains, across a membrane.

The rate of ultrafiltration (N_{UF}) depends on three factors [28]:

$$N_{UF} = T \times \overline{C}_B \times Q_f$$

21

THE STAGES OF CHRONIC RENAL FAILURE

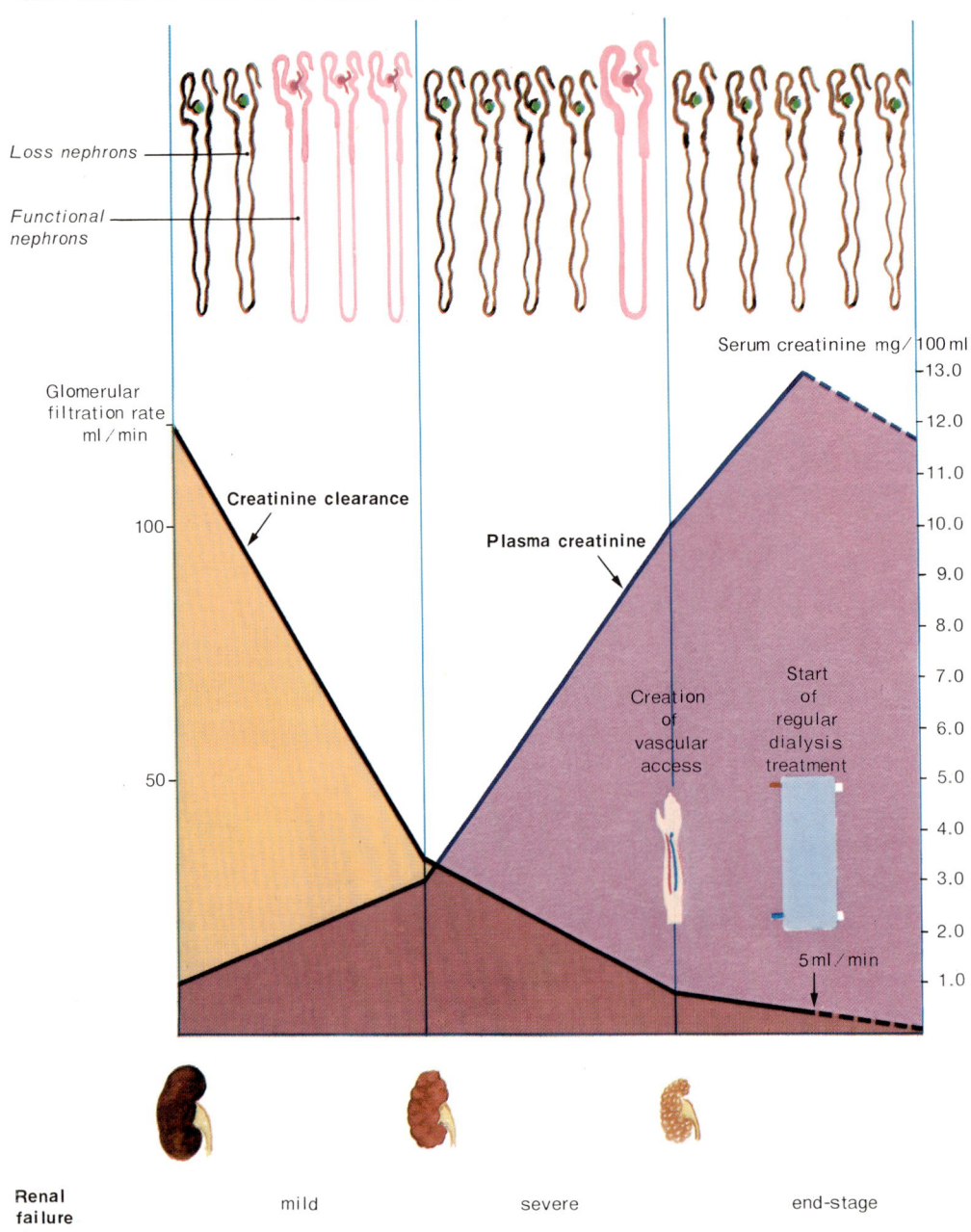

3.3.1 The sieving coefficient (T) of a membrane for a given solute is the relationship between the concentration of the solute in the ultrafiltrate and its simultaneous concentration in the blood (UF/P). For low molecular weight solutes, T equals 1, whatever membrane is used. With solutes of increasing molecular weights, T decreases progressively but depending on the nature of the membrane. When using Cuprophan T decreases to 0.60 for vitamin B_{12} (M W = 1,355 daltons) and to 0.32 for inulin (M W = 5,200 daltons). When using polyacrylonitrile, T decreases only to 0.94 for vitam B_{12} and to 0.78 for inulin. Thus, the latter membrane exhibits a higher convective transfer rate than Cuprophan® for middle and high molecular weight solutes [30], resembling performances of human glomerular basement membrane (Fig. 5).

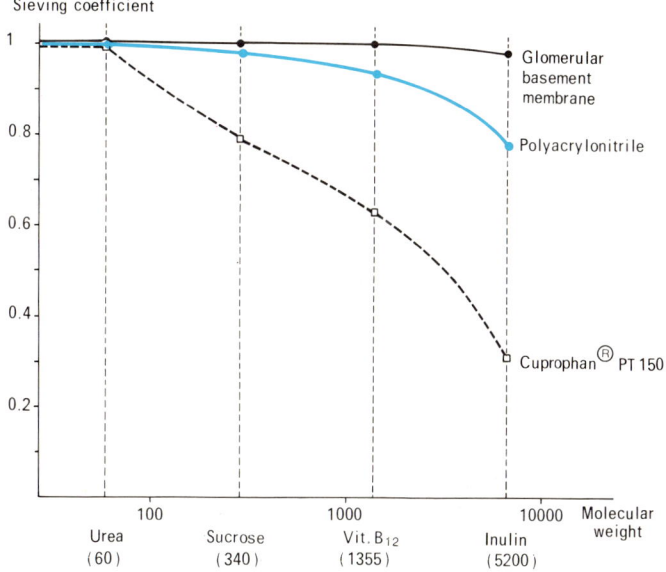

Fig. 5 - Sieving coefficient (T) of glomerular basal membrane (GBM), as compared to Cuprophan® or polyacrylonitrile membranes, for increasing molecular weight solutes.

3.3.2. The mean solute concentration of the blood ($\overline{C}_B$)

3.3.3. The solvent filtration rate, or ultrafiltration rate, (Q_f) depends on the effective surface area and hydraulic permeability of the membrane, as well as on transmembrane hydrostatic pressure.

— *Effective transmembrane pressure* is the algebraic sum of the mean positive pressure in the blood circuit, plus the mean pressure (often negative or nil) in the dialysate circuit, minus the osmotic pressure of the proteins in the blood circuit (25 to 30 mmHg).

— *Hydraulic permeability* is a physical property of a given membrane defining its capacity to transfer a solvent in a given length of time. Given equal transmembrane pressure, the ultrafiltration rate of acrylonitrile, methylacrylate or cellulose acetate membranes is far superior to that of Cuprophan® or polycarbonate membranes [31] (Fig. 6).

In conclusion, ultrafiltration, or convection, has two very different effects. On the one hand, it removes solvent, that is, plasma water, the amount of which can be adjusted to the requirements of each patient. On the other hand, ultrafiltration removes solutes contained in the plasma ultrafiltrate, according to the individual seiving coefficient of each (pl. 6).

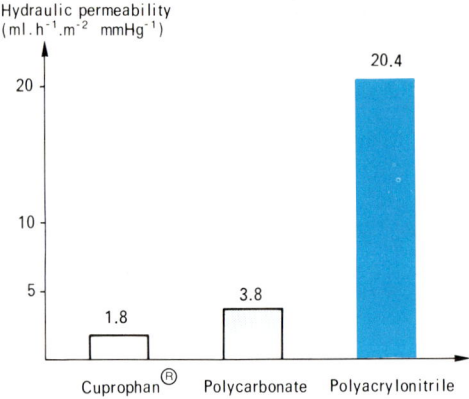

Fig. 6 - Compared hydraulic permeability of Cuprophan®, polyacrylonitrile and polycarbonate membranes.

The respective importance of ultrafiltration and diffusion varies considerably according to the molecular weight of solutes. Diffuse transfer predominates convective transport for small molecules, while higher molecular weight solutes move accross the membrane principally by convection.

3.4. Flow rates and pressure

The dialyzer exerts internal resistance to blood flow. This resistance is greater as the blood compartment is longer and the thickness of the blood film is less. The result is a pressure drop (ΔP) when the blood crosses the dialyzer. This pressure drop increases with the blood flow rate according to the law of Poiseuille [28]:

$$\Delta P = 12\mu \frac{L}{nlH^3} \times Q_B$$

This equation applies to all rectangular channels: μ represents blood viscosity, n the number of compartments, Q_B the blood flow rate and L, l and H the dimensions of the blood compartment (Fig. 7a). For cylindrical compartments (hollow-fiber dialyzers), the equation is the following:

$$P = 128\mu \frac{L}{n\pi D^4} Q_B$$

where D is the diameter of a fiber (Fig. 7b).

It results that coil dialyzers, which are composed of one or two very long blood compartments wound into a coil, have the highest pressure drop. Parallel plate or hollow-fiber dialyzers, on the other hand, have a pressure drop which is only slight or nil. In coil dialyzers, the blood compartment resistance augments with increasing flow rates, inducing varying ultrafiltration rates which are often difficult to regulate. In parallel plate or hollow-fiber dialyzers the pressure drop is little changed with increased blood flow and ultrafiltration remains stable and predictable.

The *blood flow rate* has a large effect on the dialysance of low molecular weight solutes. In contrast, it is less important or negligible for high molecular weight solutes provided blood flow rate exceeds 50 ml/min. Thus, the removal of middle molecules cannot be greatly enhanced by increasing the blood flow rate, whereas a flow rate of at least 200 ml/min. is required for the removal of urea, creatinine, or other low molecular weight toxins.

Similarly, the *dialysate flow rate* greatly affects the elimination of low molecular weight solutes, whereas above a flow rate of 150 ml/min., the dialysance of high molecular weight solutes hardly increases (Fig. 8).

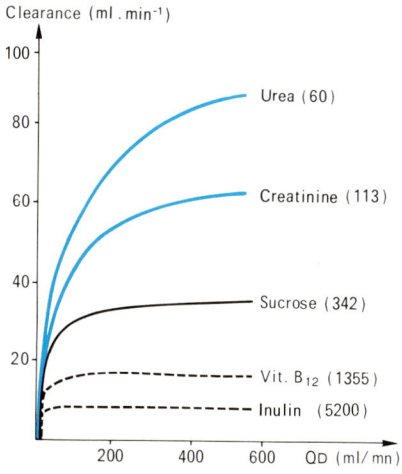

Fig. 8 - Relationship between dialysate flow and dialyzer clearance according to solute molecular weight (Kiil standard, Cuprophan® PT 150).

3.5. Evaluating dialyzer performance

The capacity of a dialyzer to remove solute and water must be measurable in order to be able to predict its performance and to compare the performances of various dialyzers [27,32]

Mass transfer of a given solute can be expressed by the clearance or by the dialysance of the dialyzer for that solute.

ENDOCRINE FUNCTIONS OF THE KIDNEY

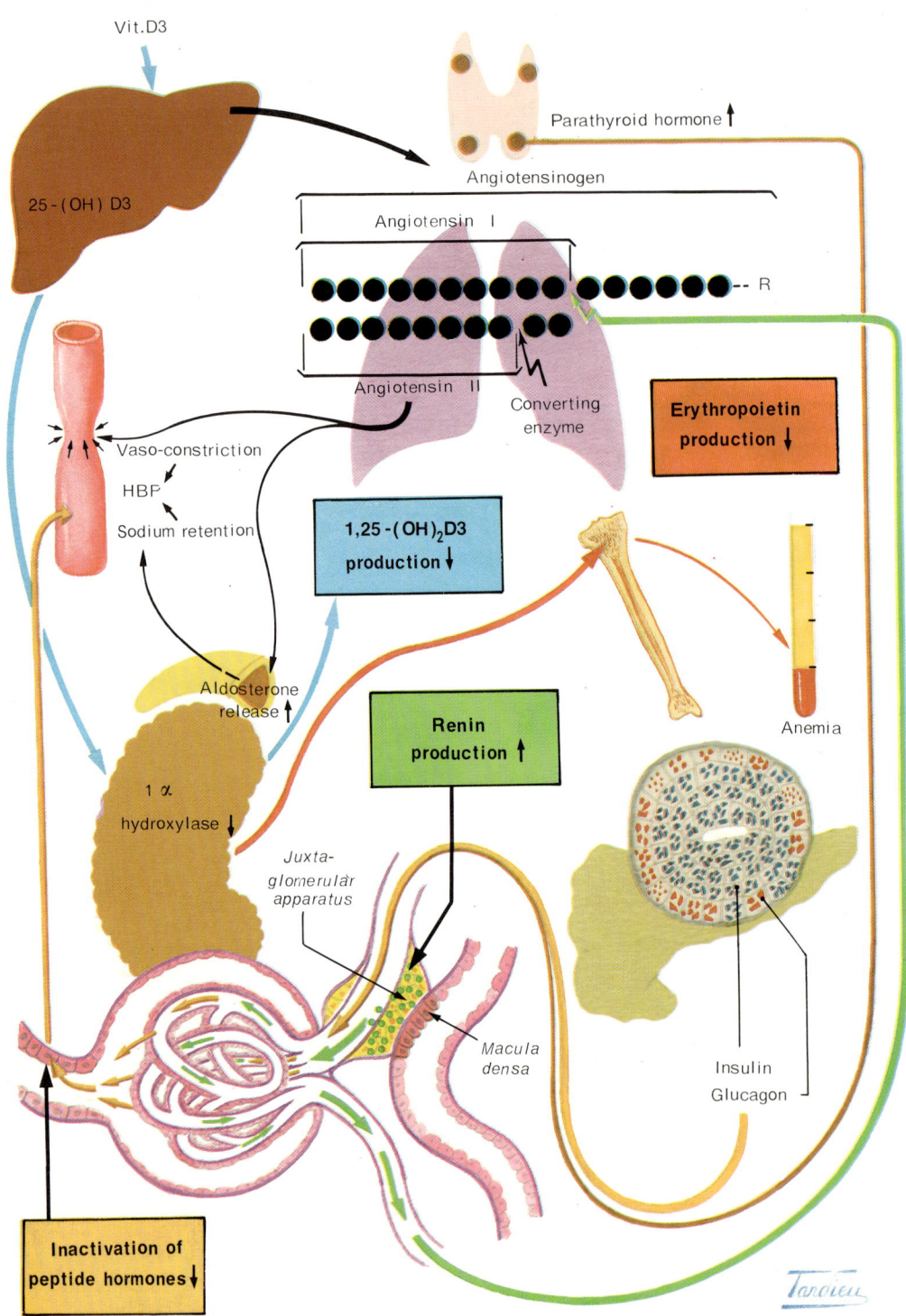

The clearance (Cl) of a dialyzer is the relationship between the mass transfer of a given solute (N) and its concentration in the blood on entering the dialyzer (C_{Bi}), or:

$$Cl = \frac{N}{C_{Bi}} = Q_B \frac{(C_{Bi} - C_{Bo})}{C_{Bi}}$$

The dialysance (D) of a dialyzer is the relationship between the blood and the dialysis fluid on entering the dialyzer ($C_{Bi} - C_{Di}$), or:

$$D = \frac{N}{(C_{Bi} - C_{Di})} = Q_B \frac{(C_{Bi} - C_{Bo})}{(C_{Bi} - C_{Di})}$$

In single-pass dialysis, C_{Di} is nil and dialysance is equal to clearance, so either measurement can be used to evaluate performance. However, only dialysance should be used in other cases, such as coil dialyzers with dialysate recirculation and all systems using closed circuit dialysis.

IV — HEMODIALYSIS EQUIPMENT

The technology involved in hemodialysis equipment has made great strides since 1960, largely thanks to constant cooperation among physicians and engineers. The equipment has become easier to use, with industrial manufacture of ready-to-use components. Safety has been increased with automatic monitoring devices. And, lastly, the length of dialysis time has been cut by better dialyzer performance and new synthetic membranes.

The dialysis equipment itself includes a dialyzer, a dialysate delivery system, and monitoring devices. We will discuss the main characteristics of the principal types in use today.

4.1. Dialyzers

A dialyzer is composed of a dialysis membrane and supporting structures. Most dialyzers in use today can be grouped into three types (plate 7):

4.1.1. Coil dialyzers

One or two flattened tubes of Cuprophan® are wound transversally around a cylindrical support, with a supporting screen. This design provoques much resistance to blood and dialysate flow. The dialysate flow rate must be very high, around 20 to 30 l/min. [33]. The pressure drop in the blood compartment is very high, requiring the use of an occlusive blood pump and provoking mandatory ultrafiltration. Ultrafiltration is difficult to regulate since it varies with blood pressure and flow [34]. The advantages of coil dialyzers are their good performance and their ease of use. Their disadvantages are a high incidence of membrane rupture because of the high pressure required to overcome the resistance of the blood circuit, and the difficulty of regulating ultrafiltration.

4.1.2. Parallel-plate dialyzers

Parallel-plate dialyzers are composed of a number (2 or more) of parallel rectangular compartments which are separated by rigid support structures giving little compliance, i.e. low deformability with pressure variation. Their pressure drop is low. The extracorporeal blood volume is lower than that of coil dialyzers, and the ultrafiltration rate is more predictable and easy to regulate.

The first parallel-plate dialyzers were composed of two large plates and had to be assembled before use, which was a time-consuming process. The original *Kiil* « standard » had longitudinal channels for dialysate flow [35]. Its size was reduced when *multipoint* support structures were introduced, which increased dialysate turbulence and thus reduced RD[36]. Later, *multiple plate* dialyzers were manufactured; they are presterilized and ready for use. Their performance is comparable to that of coil dialyzers but ultrafiltration is easier to regulate and there is less risk of membrane rupture [37].

4.1.3. Hollow-fiber dialyzers

Hollow-fiber dialyzers are composed of a group of 10,000 to 15,000 hollow fibers (capillaries), with an internal diameter of about 200 microns. The membrane is made of

Cuprophan® or cellulose acetate. Its compliance is very low. In theory, this structure is optimal: extracorporeal blood volume below 150 ml and blood film diameter less than 100 microns for a dialysis surface of 1 m² are the best of any dialyzer [38]. Blood compartment pressure drop is low and ultrafiltration is easy to regulate. Its easiness of use and its performances equal those of parallel-plate and coil dialyzers. However, a major disadvantage is that coagulation frequently occurs within the fibers. This decreases dialysis efficiency and blood restitution.

4.2. Dialysate delivery systems and monitoring devices

4.2.1. Delivery systems

The dialysis fluid is prepared by diluting a concentrated solution with treated water (pl. 8).

It can be made manually in a tank. This is the simplest system, but it requires a space-consuming installation. The most commonly used delivery systems today are mechanical devices in which the proper dialysate concentration is prepared by a proportioning pump. This method is easy to use and takes little space, but it requires an additional monitoring system to verify that the dialysis fluid is always at the proper concentration.

Dialysate delivery systems can provide dialysate fluid for one patient or for a number of posts.

Collective delivery system is the most economical, but it has two disadvantages. Firstly, it implies that all patients are dialyzed against an identical dialysate electrolyte concentration; if the composition of the dialysate is improper, the risk of accident is multiplied by the number of posts served by the system. Secondly, if the system breaks down, a whole dialysis center may be paralyzed.

Individual delivery system provide the possibility of individualizing the dialysate composition for each patient. It also limits the risk of accidents, but it is more expensive.

In a *single-pass* system, the amount of dialysate used during a 6-hour dialysis is approximately 200 liters. This quantity can be reduced by using a *closed circuit*. The Rhodial 75® uses 75 liters per dialysis [31]. The Redy® machine uses a small amount of dialysate which is regenerated in the circuit by passing through an adsorptive cartridge [39]. This method is costly, but has the advantage of being portable (plate 9).

4.2.2. Monitoring devices

Monitoring devices are used to verify continually the composition of the dialysate and to detect any abnormal occurrence in the blood or dialysate circuit (plate 10).

- **Monitoring of the blood circuit**

The basic device is a manometer which continuously registers the *pressure of the return blood circuit,* below the dialyzer. It is connected to a device which automatically halts the blood pump, thus stopping blood flow. Auditory and visual alarms are also a part of this system. An alarm sounds whenever venous pressure drops, usually reflecting a blood leak in the dialyzer, or when it rises because of increased resistance in the circuit, with the risk of membrane rupture.

Two additional alarm systems are useful. One is *blood leak detector.* It, too, can stop the blood pump if hemoglobin is detected in the dialysate. The second alarm is an *air detector* at the bubble trap on the venous return tubing. This alarm also stops the blood pump and, ideally, should be connected to an electromagnetic clamp which will stop the return flow. Both these monitoring devices have visual and auditory alarms.

- **Monitoring of the dialysate fluid**

    Dialysate control includes the following devices:
    — a *resistivimeter* which continually checks dialysate osmolality;
    — a *thermometer* verifying dialysate temperature, which should remain around 38°C. Any divergence from the set limits sets off visual and auditory alarms and puts the dialysate fluid into by-pass.

    Dialysate flow should be continuously measured by a flowmeter, which can be adjusted to the desired flow. Similarly, the *pressure of the dialysate circuit* is continuously controlled by a manometer. Any divergence will set off an alarm and stop the dialysate circulation pump. The pressure in the dialysate circuit should adjusted independently of that of the dialysate flow. Pressure in the dialysate circuit is adjusted as to obtain the rate of ultrafiltration desired.

4.3. The dialysate fluid

The dialysate fluid is a nonsterile aqueous solution with an electrolyte composition near that of normal extracellular fluid. It contains none of the solutes which should be eliminated from the blood of the hemodialyzed patient (urea, creatinine and other waste products of nitrogen metabolism). Its electrolyte composition is designed to correct the disorders which develop between dialyses. It should be noted that the electrolyte composition of extracellular fluid is somewhat different from that of plasma: interstitial fluids contain almost no proteins and their chloride concentration is about 10 % more than that of plasma.

4.3.1. The composition of the dialysate fluid

The standard dialysate fluid used in various centers is very similar. As an example, below are the solute concentrations used at Necker Hospital, expressed as mEq/l of diluted solution:

Cations		Anions	
Sodium	145	Chloride	114
Potassium	2	Acetate	38
Calcium	3.5	(Glucose)	0
Magnesium	1.5		
	152		152

In some cases, modifications of this standard dialysate may be necessary.

— *Sodium*: initially used dialysates had a low sodium concentration, often below 140 mEq/l. Those now used have a higher sodium content, of approximately 145 mEq/l. This is in better equilibrium with the extracellular fluid and avoids sodium depletion, responsible for cramps during dialysis sessions.

— *Potassium*: the potassium concentration permits the removal of potassium which accumulates between dialyses. However, a potassium-rich dialysate (up to 3 or even 4 mEq/l) may be necessary when potassium depletion at the end of a dialysis session provokes cardiac arrhythmias.

DIFFUSION (OR CONDUCTION) TRANSFER

Pl. 4

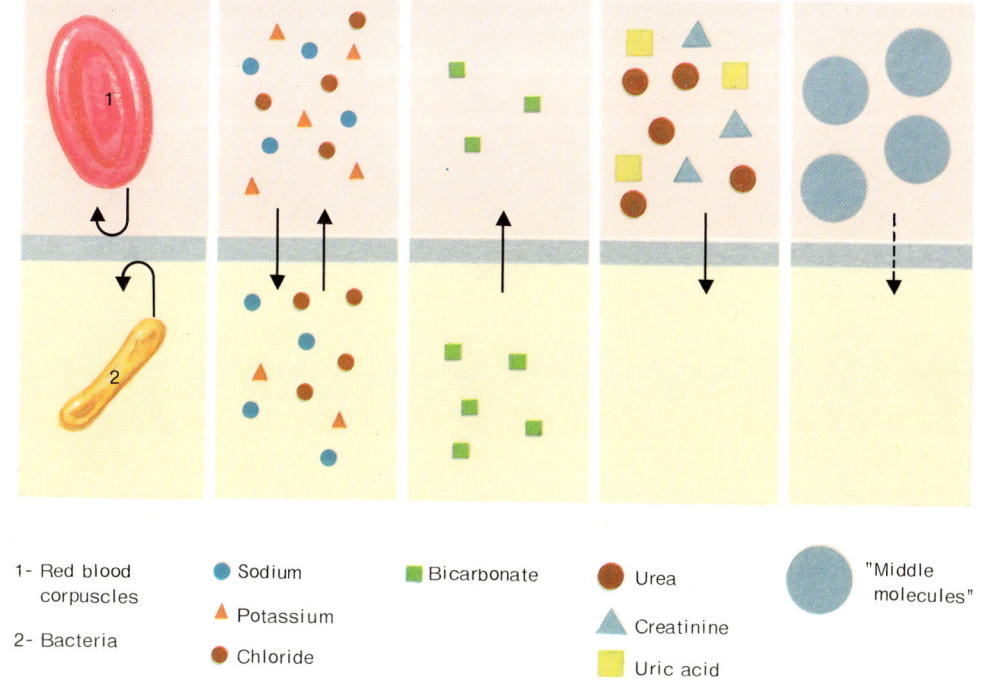

Principles of diffusion transfer across dialysis membranes

Schematic representation of resistance opposed to diffusion transfer in a dialyzer

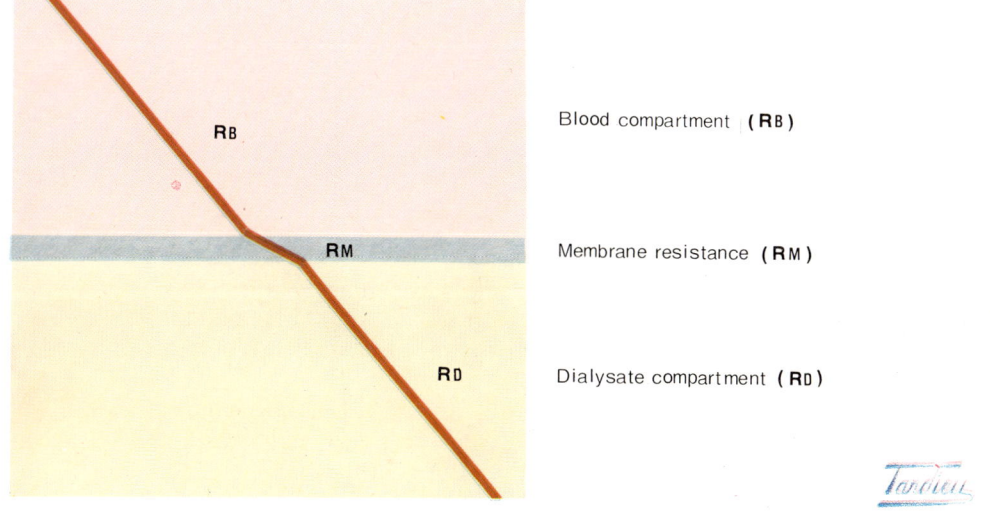

— *Calcium* : calcium concentration of the dialysate varies among centers between 60 to 75 mg/l. It appears that the concentration which brings optimal calcium transfer from the dialysate to the patient, without inducing excessive hypercalcemia, is about 70 mg/l [40,41].

4.3.2. Preparation of dialysate concentrates

Since the amount of dialysate required for a single dialysis session is large, the dialysate is prepared industrially in concentrated form and presented in 10-liter containers. The usual concentrates should be diluted 35 to 40 times : this concentration corresponds to the limit of mineral salt solubility. Three points should be particularly noted :

— *Concentration of sodium* : when the dialysate is prepared with soft water, a lower concentration of sodium should be used (softened water contains about 5 mEq/l of sodium, for a calcium exchange of 100 mg/l).

— *Glucose* : glucose is usually not included in the dialysate in order to avoid bacterial growth. However, for diabetic patients, a dialysate containing 1 to 2 g/l of glucose should be used.

— *Sodium acetate* : since the bicarbonate ion precipitates in the presence of calcion ions, its precursor, acetate, is used in the concentrated solution [42]. Nevertheless, in patients with liver cell dysfunction, acetate may not be metabolized quickly enough by the liver. In this case, it is preferable to use a concentrate which contains no acetate and to add the desired amount of sodium bicarbonate to the concentrate immediately before use.

4.3.3. Water treatment

In most cases, city water, as it comes out of the tap, cannot be used for preparing the dialysis bath because of its high content of mineral and organic substances, which even vary from day to day. The main **undesirable substances** are [43] :

— *Calcium* : a high concentration of calcium, often over 100 mg/l, has caused acute hypercalcemia (« hard-water syndrome ») when the dialysate was prepared with untreated water [44]. The water which is used must therefore contain no calcium, and the required concentration of calcium ions must be added to it.

— *Nitrates and nitrites* : they are the result of bacterial contamination of the water and can cause acute methemoglobinemia. They are found especially in rural areas.

— *Chloramines* : these are oxidizing compounds used in antibacterial treatment of city water. They can cause acute hemolysis.

— *Copper* : the copper content in water can come from water pipes, but it can also be contained in the water itself. Excessive copper concentration can cause hemolysis.

— *Sulfates* : their excessive concentration brings digestive disorders such as nausea and vomiting.

— *Fluoride* : fluoride may cause disturbances in bone mineralization.

— *Aluminum* : water aluminum can accumulate in the blood and certain organs, notably the brain. This causes severe encephalopathy [45].

— *Pyrogens* : they are usually composed of toxins resulting from bacterial contamination.

— *Iron* : high iron content harms the dialysis and water treatment equipment.

— *Suspended particles* : they can obstruct pipes and tubing in the equipment.

Proper treatment is necessary to rid the water of these impurities, or to lower their concentration to within acceptable limits. Comty et al. suggest that the water used for preparation of the dialysis bath should have no more than the following maximum concentrations of these substances [43]:

Substances	Maximum tolerated concentrations
Calcium	0
Magnesium	0
Iron-Manganese	0
Fluoride	0.2 mg/l
Copper	0
Sulfates	100 mg/l
Nitrates	2 mg/l
Chloramines	0.1 mg/l
Pyrogens	0
Suspended particles	<5 microns in diameter

There are many **methods for treating water**. According to the characteristics of the water available in any given center, several methods often have to be used simultaneously.

The main methods for treating city water are following (plate 11).

A *sedimentation filter* removes particles larger than 5 microns in diameter. It is an indispensable first step in preparing the water for dialysis.

When iron concentration in city water is above 0.3 mg/l, an *oxidizing filter* which fixes iron should be added at this step.

Activated *charcoal filters* remove free chloride, chloramines, organic substances and pyrogens, which are not removed by exchange resins.

Water softeners contain cation resins which exchange Ca^{++} and Mg^{++} ions in water against Na^+ ions. Thus, when the calcium concentration of water is initially 100 mg/l, its sodium content is increased by about 5 mEq/l of sodium. Water softeners also remove iron, manganese and aluminum. When only the calcium and magnesium content of the water needs to be corrected, treatment by water softener alone suffices. This is a particularly good method for home dialysis, but the resins must be regularly regenerated and a careful rinsing must follow in order to avoid hypercalcemia or sodium overload.

Total deionization or demineralization consists of simultaneous use of cation exchange resins (removing sodium, calcium and magnesium) and anionic resins (removing sulfates, chloride and nitrates). Their operating cost is high because the resins must often be regenerated.

Reverse osmosis is a physical process, partially demineralizing the water [46]. It is based on ultrafiltration under high pressure against an osmotic gradient. It can be used as a step preceding that of deionization, but this method has also proven costly.

In summary, for home dialysis filtration plus softening of the water is usually sufficient, as long as it is properly performed.

In dialysis centers an appropriate combination of these methods should be used, based on the mean composition of the available water. The water composition should be regularly checked.

STRUCTURE OF DIALYSIS MEMBRANES

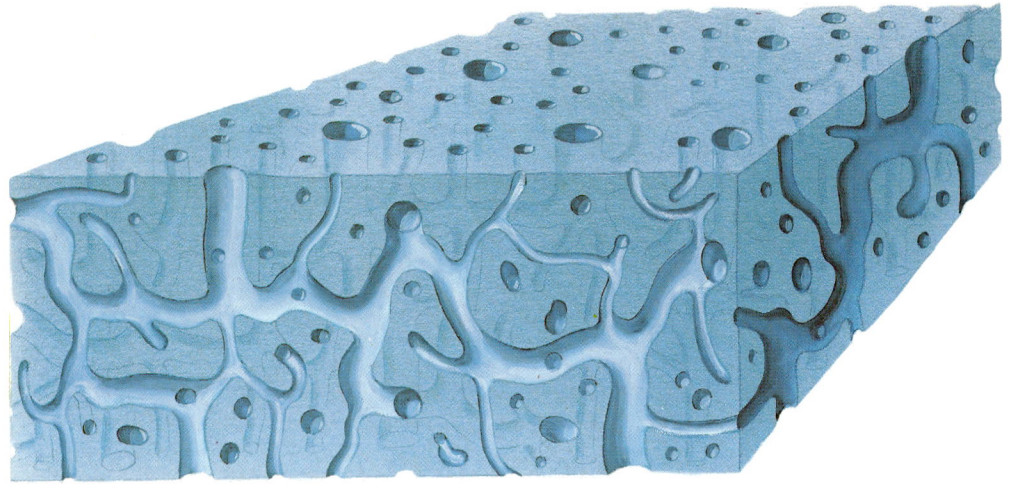

Artist's representation of "channels" of various sizes crossing through a membrane.

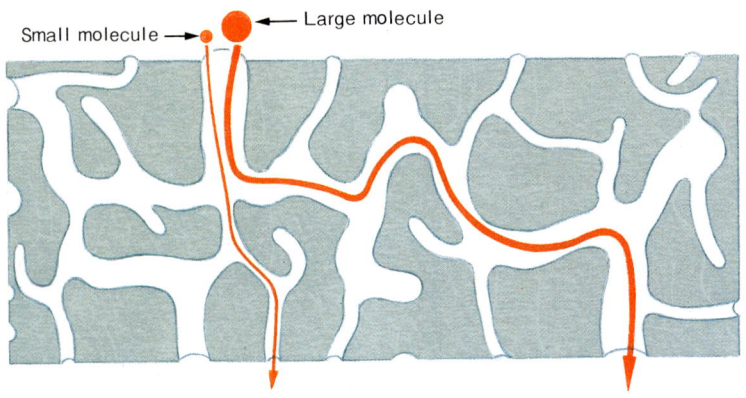

Artist's impression of large and small molecules crossing the membrane at different speeds.

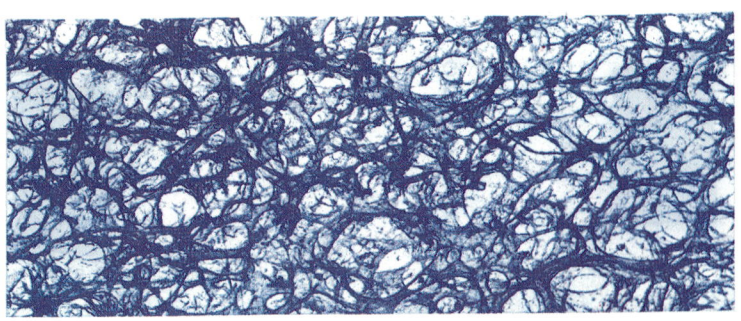

Electron microscopy of a cellulose membrane: in fact, the "channels" are formed by interlacing cellulose fibers.

4.4. The special case of hemofiltration (pl. 12)

Hemofiltration is a new method of waste product removal. It uses exclusively convective solute transfer through membranes which have a high hydraulic permeability and high transmittance coefficient for « middle molecules »[47].

This method is aimed at removing a large amount of « middle molecules » and higher molecular weight solutes, while also removing a sufficient amount of lower weight solutes. The membranes are cellulosic, such as Amicon® XM 50[48] or are made of polyacrylonitrile [49,50]. With the latter membrane, using a surface area of 1 m² and hydrostatic transmembrane pressure of 300 mmHg, ultrafiltration flow is about 70 ml/min., or 20 liters in 5 hours [50]. The water and electrolytes which are removed have to be continually replaced with a sterile isotonic solution, such as that used in peritoneal dialysis.

This method is still in clinical experimentation, but it seems very promising. Interestingly, it closely reflects the glomerular function in the human kidney and would seem to lend itself to future miniaturization. In addition, and for reasons as yet unknown, hemofiltration has been said to control arterial hypertension particularly well and to correct the hypertriglyceridemia often found in uremic patients [49]. However, in its present state of development, the functioning cost of hemofiltration is higher than that of hemodialysis.

4.5. Dialyzer performance (pl. 13)

For clinical purposes, dialyzer performance is expressed as clearance. To determine clearance, three factors are separately assessed : 1) the removal of low molecular weight solutes such as urea and creatinine ; 2) the removal of « middle molecules » such as vitamin B_{12} (MW = 1,355) ; and 3) the ultrafiltration rate [51].

As seen on the table I (p. 47), the performance of almost all Cuprophan dialyzers using a membrane surface of 1 m² is nearly identical, whether coil, parallel plate or hollow-fiber. For purposes of comparison, we have indicated the performance of dialyzers using membranes having high permeability for « middle molecules » : polyacrylonitrile [31], polycarbonate [52], and polymethacrylate. The indicated values have been measured in vitro in the Necker Hospital dialysis laboratory.

V — VASCULAR ACCESS

B.H. Scribner was the first to create an arteriovenous shunt in 1960 [53]. It was the first permanent means of easy access to the blood for the treatment of chronic uremia. Since then, the technique has been perfected, especially with the arteriovenous fistula suggested by Cimino and Brescria in 1966 [54]. Other techniques are now also available but are less frequently used [55].

5.1. The main types of vascular access (pl. 14)

In order to avoid side-effects which might be detrimental to the heart, vascular access is usually created on a medium-size artery, such as the radial artery. Sometimes, however, a larger artery must be used.

5.1.1. Arteriovenous shunts

The *Quinton-Scribner shunt* consists of two Teflon® cannulae, placed in the radial artery at the wrist and in a vein of the lower arm[56]. Each cannula is connected to a piece of Silastic® tubing, and the two tubes are exteriorally connected by a removable Teflon® component. This shunt canal also be placed between the posterior tibial artery and the internal saphenous vein, or, generally speaking, between any peripheral artery and a neighboring vein. It can be put into place rapidly using only local anesthesia and can be used immediately. Unfortunately, thrombosis occurs frequently, as does infection at the points where the Silastic® tubing emerges from the skin.

The *Buselmeier shunt* is a U-shaped arteriovenous shunt having two outlets which are each plugged with Teflon obturators when not in use [57]. The risk of infection by handling is thereby reduced. However, the longevity of this device does not seem to exceed that of the classic Scribner shunt.

The *Thomas shunt* is composed of two Silastic® cannulae connected laterally by a Dacron® applique to femoral vessels [58]. The Silastic element is encapsulated in Dacron velvet at skin exit sites, serving as a mechanical barrier to infection. Thrombosis is infrequent, because of the high flow rate of femoral vessels. However, the risk of thrombosis or infection remains and is serious because of the proximal location of the shunt.

5.1.2. Internal fistulae

The *Cimino-Brescia arteriovenous fistula* is the type of vascular access most used today. In 85 percent of cases, it is the initial vascular access used. The fistula is usually made between the radial artery at the wrist and the superficial radial vein by side-to-side, or better, end-to-side anastomosis. The fistula can also be created at a more proximal location, for instance at the origin of the radial artery.

Since healing and development of the fistula require several weeks or months, this vascular access cannot be used immediately. However, its advantages are great. Risks of infection and thrombosis are much less than with external shunts, and its longevity is superior.

In some cases, it may be impossible to create a fistula, due to insufficient development of the venous network or previous multiple venous ligatures. Then other solutions must be found, such as grafting an arteriovenous by-pass.

5.1.3. Arteriovenous grafts

The graft (which may be autologous, homologous, heterologous or synthetic) is inserted between an artery (radial artery at its origin, or humeral, axillary or femoral arteries), and a nearby vein. The by-pass can be curvilinear or rectilinear. Several types of grafts are used [55]:

— a *saphenous autograft*, that is, the own internal saphenous vein of the patient, removed from Scarpa's triangle. It can be placed between the humeral or radial artery and a vein at the elbow. Also, it may be sectioned and connected in situ, either to the superficial femoral artery or to the popliteal artery after its superficialization;

— a *saphenous homograft*, that is an internal saphenous vein preserved after surgical repair of varicose veins, can be used in the same manner;

— *bovine carotid grafts* are frequently used today. They are prepared by trypsic digestion to reduce antigenicity [59]. Since any number of lengths and calibres are available, they can be used for all types of grafting;

— *synthetic vessels*, made of Dacron® or polytetrafluoroethylen [60] have recently been proposed. Their reliability has not yet been demonstrated.

5.1.4. Arterial jump grafts

In some cases, no vein is available for internal or external anastomosis. In these rare cases an arterio-arterial by-pass can be created, for instance by subcutaneous transposition of the superficial femoral artery or a femoro-popliteal by-pass using a vascular graft, which has excellent hemodynamic tolerance.

5.1.5. Percutaneous route

In an emergency situation or in the case of temporary lack of vascular access, blood access may be made by percutaneous puncture of the femoral vein at the inguinal fold. This technique can be used several times if necessary, but deep hematoma can result.

5.2. Complications involved in vascular access

Vascular access entails the risk of local complications which can threaten their longevity. There can also be hemodynamic repercussions [61].

5.2.1. Local complications

Infection is more frequent with external shunts than with fistulae. However, in a fistula, an infection may be undetected for a longer time. A venous infection carries the risk of bacterial spread and development of metastatic septic localizations. Infection can also cause hemorrhage by suture or cannula release. The existence of infection often requires removal of the shunt or of the fistula. It follows that strict hygiene must be observed with regard to cannula exit sites, to connection and disconnection of shunts and to needle insertion or removal in fistulae.

Thrombosis is particularly frequent in arteriovenous shunts using synthetic material. Clotting of the *Scribner shunt* can be alleviated by aspiration of clots with a thin catheter.

PRINCIPLES OF ULTRAFILTRATION

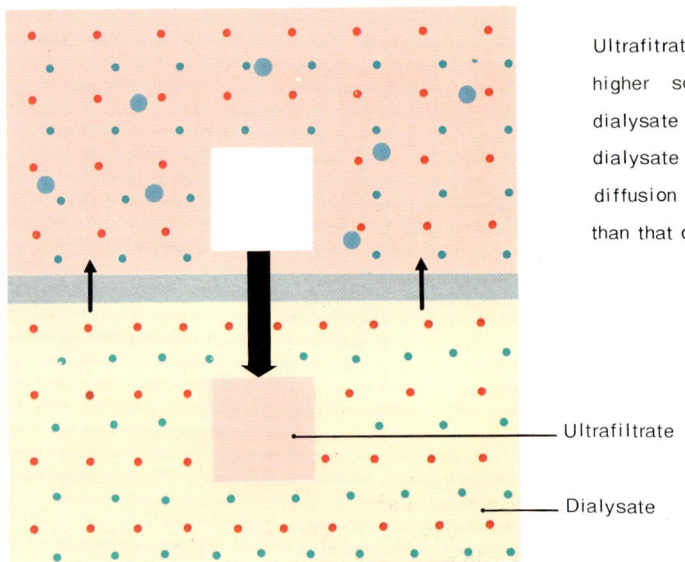

Ultrafitration against **osmotic gradient**. The higher solute concentration within the dialysate carries **water** from plasma to dialysate (with the condition that solute diffusion through the membrane is slower than that of water molecules).

— Ultrafiltrate

— Dialysate

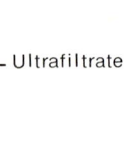

Ultrafiltration through **hydrostatic pressure gradient,** creating a simultaneous transfer of **solvent** (plasma water) and **solutes** (according to their sieving coefficient) out of the plasma.

— Ultrafiltrate

When this manœuver is only partly successful, it can be complemented by local injection of fibrinolytic agents. No more than 2 ml of heparin solution should be injected into the artery during these maneuvers, in order to minimize the risk of *retrograde arterial embolism* [62]. If coagulation in the shunt is repeated, a fistulography should be made. It will often show a stenosis of the vein below the cannula (« jet lesion »). Repair consists of placing the venous cannula just above the affected zone or, if this is not possible, in another vein.

Declotting of *internal fistulae* is more difficult and is usually impossible for small-size distal fistulae. Arteriovenous grafts, which usually have a larger diameter, can often be cleared by a Fogarty catheter. The veno-venous anastomosis should almost always be repaired at the same time. The desobstruction can also be attempted with the aid of fibrinolytic agents, but close surveillance of the patient must be maintained. If it is successful, *fistulography* should be performed to seek the cause of the thrombosis : stenosis of the vein below the fistula, graft folding, or bad positioning of the anastomosis. Any of these causes should be surgically corrected. *Aneurysm* of the arterialized vein occurs only in internal fistulae. It can be favoured by frequent use of the same puncture point. When there is risk of rupture or an important esthetic reason, the aneurysm should be corrected by surgery.

5.2.2. Hemodynamic consequences

External, distal shunts, which have a flow rate of about 250 ml/min., and fistulae with a moderate flow rate, are usually well-tolerated by the heart. On the contrary, arteriovenous anastomoses with a high flow rate can affect local or cardiac hemodynamics.

The *local effect* is a « vascular steal » syndrome. It mostly occurs when the artery supplying the fistula is too large, the arteriovenous anastomosis is too wide and the collateral circulation is reduced because of parietal caclcifications or ligature of the peripheral arteries. The vascular steal syndrome is reflected by cramps and painful paresthesias in the distal part of the limbs, particularly when making an effort. Occasionally, peripheric ischemia can provoque gangrene [61].

The *effect on the heart* is detectable only for internal arteriovenous fistula with excessive development, or for arteriovenous grafts inserted on proximal vessels, when the blood flow rate reaches 1 to 3 liters per minute [63]. In such cases, high-output heart failure can be improved or corrected after surgical reduction of the fistula blood flow rate.

In conclusion, the creation of the vascular access is very important, for upon it depends the patient's survival through many years of dialysis. It should be done by a well-trained surgeon who is acquainted with vascular microsurgery and is interested in performing this type of surgery.

VI. ORGANIZATION OF DIALYSIS TREATMENT

Chronic hemodialysis can be performed in a center or at home. The latter has the advantage of greater independance and aids the professional rehabilitation of the patient. The initiation of hemodialysis should be preceded by appropriate preparation, including the creation of good vascular access. The protocol to assure efficient dialysis, capable of maintaining the patient in good general state without uremic complications, should be established for each case [51].

6.1. Modalities of chronic hemodialysis

Hemodialysis was initially performed only in hospitals. Very soon, Scribner's group developed the concept of home dialysis [64] which was subsequently to develop, especially in United Kingdom [65].

6.1.2. Center dialysis.
The optimum size of hemodialysis units seems to be 8 to 10 posts, allowing treatment of 20 to 30 patients. It is preferable that the hemodialysis unit be a part of a hospital organization for easy handling of the medical or surgical problems that can confront hemodialyzed patients. Theoretically, center dialysis should be provided for patients who do not have a family setting that would allow home dialysis and to those in poor general status or of high risk.

6.1.3. Home dialysis
is the best solution for cooperative and emotionally stable patients, with family support (spouse or parents) and adequate housing. Training usually takes 6 to 8 weeks. Material considerations such as living conditions rarely are a limiting factor for home dialysis because of the relatively small size of present machines. Similarly, the social or cultural level of the patient seems to have little effect on whether the training is successful [66]. The main factor determining success or failure appears to be the motivation of the patient and his family, although self-dialysis has proven to be possible. The chief advantage of home dialysis is a greater freedom in the choice of dialysis times, which allows better professional and family rehabilitation.

6.1.4. Self care or limited-care
dialysis can replace home dialysis when either housing or family surroundings are not sufficient for home dialysis [67]. The units may be located either within or outside of a hospital. Patients perform their own dialyses, and a technician is responsible for upkeep of the equipment.

With the present reduction in the length of dialysis [68], *overnight dialysis is* progressively being replaced, both for hospital and home treatment [65], by *evening dialysis sessions* [6].

6.2. Preparation for regular dialysis treatment

When dialysis becomes necessary in a uremic patient, several preliminary steps should be carefully organized.

6.2.1. Psychological preparation of the patient

Several months before the expected initiation of hemodialysis, the patient should be informed of the need for regular dialysis treatment. The basic concept should be carefully explained, particularly the indefinite nature of the treatment unless transplantation is performed. It should be stressed that the patient's state will be so improved with dialysis that professional and family activity can remain very close to normal.

The patient and his spouse should be consulted at length when it appears that home dialysis may be possible. When home dialysis is not possible, the patient should be added to the waiting list at the center closest to his home.

Some *psychological trauma* is inevitable when the patient learns that he is faced with indefinite treatment by hemodialysis. The best means of combatting this trauma is to make the patient understand that thousands of other patients in the same situation are not only kept alive but become capable of leading a nearnormal life with dialysis. Patient associations may be a further help in facing dialysis treatment.

6.2.2. Creation of vascular access

Today, the internal arteriovenous fistula is the most common means of initial vascular access. It must be created several weeks or months before the first dialysis to allow sufficient healing and development of the fistula.

> **It is recommended that a fistula be created as soon as plasma creatinine level reaches 8,0 to 10,0 mg/100 ml, and even sooner in female, aged or diabetic patients, and patients with a poorly developed venous network.**

6.2.3. Exploration of the possibility of renal transplantation

Outside of contraindications such as age over about 50 years or anatomical disorders of the lower urinary tract, the possibility of renal transplantation should be explored [1]. This exploration includes :

— retrograde or suspubic *cystography* followed by endoscopic or surgical correction of any anomalies when possible ;

— determination of *histocompatibility* groups and search for anti-HLA antibodies, as well as registration on the waiting list of the national organization which groups transplant recipients and distributes available kidneys according to histocompatibility ;

— search within the family of the patient for a voluntary adult donor who is histocompatible and free of any renal or extrarenal disease.

In each case, it is useful to determine the *type of initial renal disease,* particularly when glomerulonephritis is involved. This is because some types of glomerulonephritis can recur on the transplanted kidney and lead to transplant failure. Any patients who have a definite contraindication to transplantation should be told of this fact and directed toward home dialysis.

6.3. Individual protocol for treatment

> **The aim of dialysis is to maintain the patient in good general status and to prevent extrarenal or metabolic complications due to uremic toxicity. This goal can be achieved by a weekly dialysis duration sufficient to eliminate toxic metabolites and to correct water and electrolyte disorders, without making the weekly dialysis time too invasive.**

Recent theoretical calculations have been made to determine the minimum weekly dialysis time for each patient, based on membrane characteristics, dialyzers used and the clinical status of the patient.

6.3.1. Criteria for adequate dialysis

> **Regular dialysis treatment may be considered adequate if the patient is in good general health, without visceral or metabolic complications, and is fully rehabilitated.**

All following criteria should be present in a patient who is adequately dialyzed [69,70]:

- good general and nutritional status,
- normal blood pressure, with or without hypotensive drugs,
- well-torelated anemia,
- absence of major disorders of phosphorus and calcium metabolism,
- absence of uremic polyneuritis,
- plasma urea and creatinine concentrations, before dialysis, in the optimal range for the type of dialysis used,
- electrolyte and plasma balance near normal,
- satisfying life and good social and professional rehabilitation.

These clinical and laboratory criteria provide only an *a posteriori* evaluation of dialysis adequacy. Theoretical criteria have been developed in an attempt to determine the dialysis protocol required in a given patient. They are based on the hypothesis of Babb and Scribner concerning the role of « middle molecules » in uremia [71]. After experimenting a number of dialysis protocols, it could be shown that polyneuritis, which is considered to be the main reflection of uremic toxicity, could be prevented when « middle molecules », expressed as vitamin B_{12} clearance, are removed at the rate of 3 ml/min, or 30 liters per week [72].

6.3.2. Individual choice of treatment

Using the known performance of various dialyzers (tabl. I p. 47), it is theoretically possible to calculate the *minimum weekly dialysis time* required [72]. It depends on three factors:

— the *patient's body weight,* which determines the volume of this urea pool: the higher roughly parallels protein intake, but it is still impossible to determine [74];

— the patient's body weight, which determines the volume of his urea pool: the higher the body weight, the greater the amount of urea to be removed through dialysis. In patients weighing under 50 kg, two dialyses per week are usually sufficient. In those weighing over 60 kg, or receiving 80 mg per day or more of proteins, three weekly dialysis sessions are needed;

— the *residual diuresis,* which plays an important role in the elimination of toxins with a molecular weight over 1 000 daltons [75]. For example, a residual diuresis of 750 ml/day corresponds to a vitamin B_{12} clearance rate of 5 liters per week: this allows reducing the weekly dialysis time in the same proportion. However, dialysis time should never be reduced in anephric or anuric patients.

Other clinical findings should indicate longer dialysis time: uncontrollable hypertension pericarditis, etc.

Some authors have proposed that dialysis time be based on these criteria and calculated by the means of computers for each patient. It should be stressed, however, that these

PRINCIPAL TYPES OF DIALYZERS

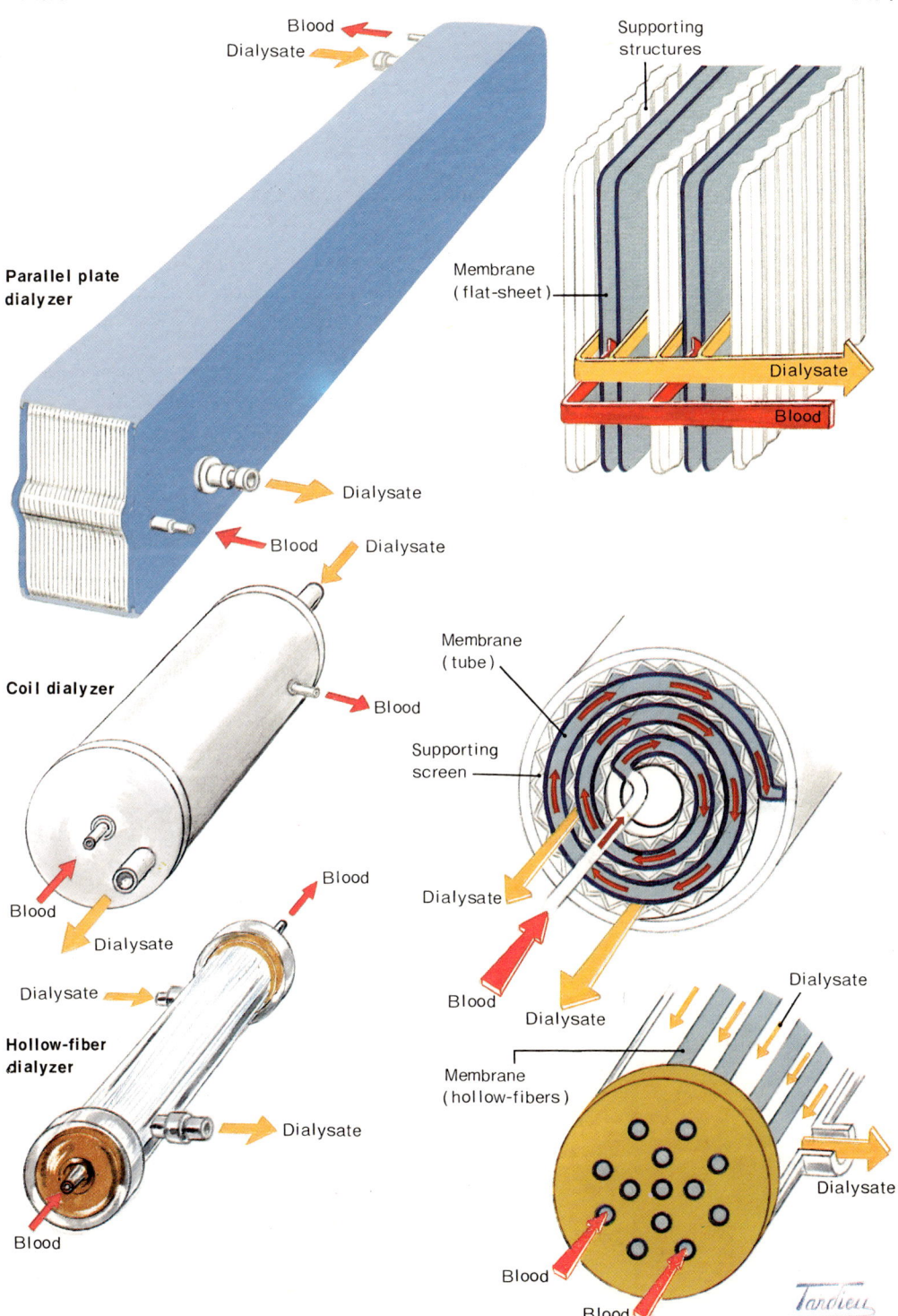

theoretical calculations are still only indicative. Semi-quantitative measurements of « middle molecule » plasma concentrations are poorly correlated with predicted values [76].

> **Thus, the adequacy of dialysis should always be verified by periodical clinical examinations.**

6.3.3. Reduction of the weekly dialysis time

In general, the average dialysis duration is 6 to 8 hours, for three to two times a week.

In order to reduce weekly dialysis time, a wish of all dialyzed patients, two methods were recently developed :

— dialyzers having membranes with a *large effective surface area*. In some hollow-fiber dialyzers, it has been raised to 1.5 m² and even 3 m² (table 1). Unfortunately, this increases extracorporeal blood volume and accelerates transfer of low molecular weight solutes, which is often poorly tolerated,

— *membranes with high permeability for « middle molecules »* such as those made of polycarbonate and polyacrylonitrile (fig. 9). The RP6®, which has a polyacrylonitrile membrane of 1 m² and is in a closed dialysate system provides sufficient dialysis for most patients in three weekly sessions of 4 hours each. Predialysis urea and creatinine concentrations are above that seen before dialysis with classic dialyzers, as a result of the use of a closed circuit, but this has no clinical manifestation.

In sum, although it would today be possible to increase dialyzer performance even more, it does not seem that each session can be less than 3 hours. When dialysis is shorter, disorders related to the imbalance of urea concentration among the various water compartments of the body appear. This *osmotic disequilibrium syndrome* is due to the fact that urea is thought to diffuse more slowly out of intracellular water, notably out of muscle and cerebral cells, than out of the interstitial space (fig. 10). The result would be water transfer into the cells, bringing on cramps, headaches and even convulsions [77]. Shorter duration dialysis also reduces removal of various uremic toxins, including middle molecules, whose removal from the intracellular compartment is slow [78].

> **It results that the rate of internal transfers within the body itself limits the possibility of reducing the length of dialysis sessions.**
>
> **In the present state of our knowledge, it does not seem advisable to attempt to reduce the duration of dialysis below three hours, three times a week,.**

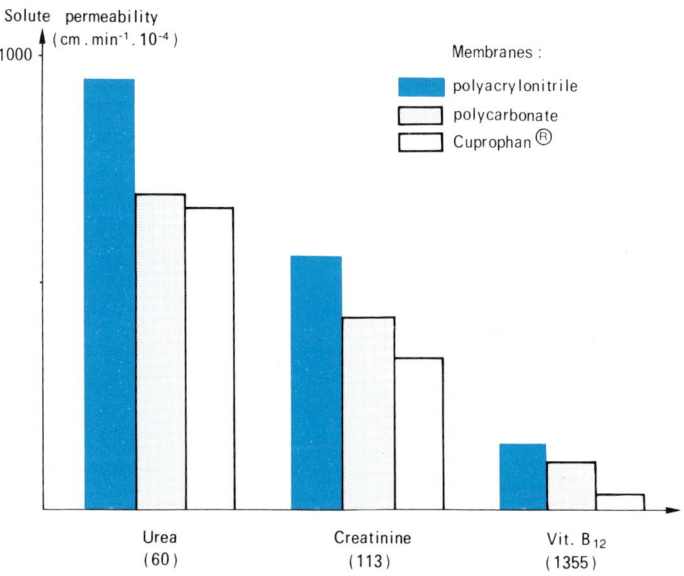

Fig. 9 - Compared solute permeability of Cuprophan®, polyacrylonitrile and polycarbonate membranes for solutes of increasing molecular weight.

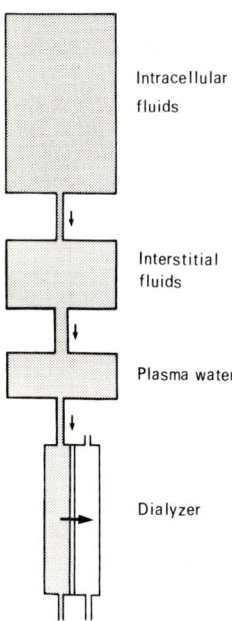

Fig. 10 - Solute transfer from intracellular compartment to dialyzer through interstitial fluids and plasma water.

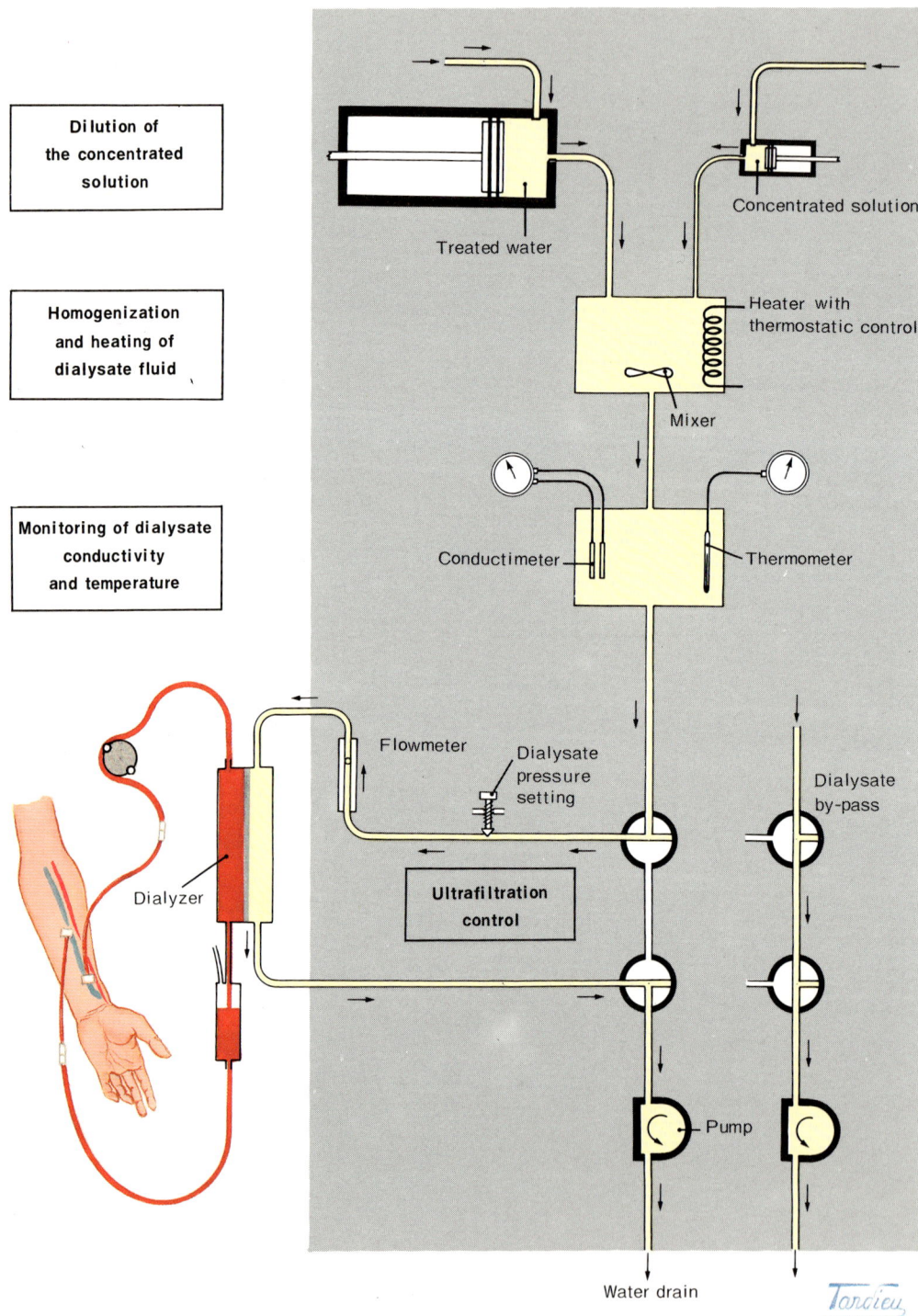

TABLE I

Performance of the main types of dialyzers

DIALYZER	MEMBRANE	ACTIVE SURFACE AREA (m²)	BLOOD VOLUME (ml)	UF ml/h mmHg	CLEARANCE (ml/mn)		
					urea	creatinine	Vit. B_{12}
Kiil	Cuprophan	1,0	400	2,5	90	68	17
Coil	Cuprophan	1,0	250	5,0	150	120	25
Parallel plate	Cuprophan	1,0	150	2,5	130	110	25
Hollow fiber	Cuprophan	1,0	90	2,5	120	110	25
Coil	Cuprophaan	1,4	300	6,5	160	140	40
Parallel plate	Cuprophan	1,4	200	3,0	150	130	40
Hollow fiber	Cellulose	2,5	200	4,0	180	150	30
Parallel plate	Acrylonitrile	1,0	150	30	140	120	60
	Polycarbonate	1,0	150	4,5	120	95	45
Hollow fiber	Methacrylate	1,0	90	27	130	110	60
	Cellulose Acetate	2,50	200	30	180	150	90

VII. PERFORMANCE AND FOLLOW-UP OF REGULAR DIALYSIS TREATEMENT

During a six-year period, with thrice weekly dialysis, nearly one thousand hemodialysis are performed in a patient. In order to assure perfect safety, the same careful monitoring must be carried out for each of these dialysis sessions.

7.1. Performance of the hemodialysis session

The first few sessions require particular precaution.

7.1.1. **The first hemodialysis sessions** should be performed in a center. The dialysis should be short, with a low dialysate flow, in order to avoid an *osmotic disequilibrium syndrome* due to an excessively rapid transfer of urea. Even with this precaution, nausea and headaches often occur.

When a *profound hypocalcemia* exists, it should first be corrected and an intravenous calcium perfusion should be maintained during the first dialysis sessions to avoid convulsions accompanying the rapid correction of acidosis [79].

Hypotensive drugs should be progressively reduced, because sodium depletion induced by the first dialyses may induce orthostatic hypotension.

Sodium and water intake should be adjusted according to residual diuresis, which tends to drop with the reduction of the osmotic load due to high urea concentration. Protein intake should be increased to reach at least 1 g/kg body weight day.

7.1.2. **Later sessions** are simpler and usually accident-free, when adequate techniques are used. The sequence in preparing and performing a dialysis session is as follows:

1. *Preparation of equipment*

A tray containing everything required for starting the dialysis session is prepared in advance (plate 15). The blood lines of the dialyzer are purged with a liter of isotonic salt solution containing 50 mg of sodium heparinate. Monitoring devices should be verified (plate 16-17).

2. *Vascular connection*

When a *fistula or an arteriovenous graft* is used, the « venous » needle for blood return to the patient is usually inserted first (plate 18). It is connected to a heparinized line, which is clamped. The « arterial » needle is then inserted, counter-current and several centimeters distal from the venous needle. It is fixed to a connecting line which is attached to the arterial line of the dialyzer. After declamping, the blood flows through the dialyzer and returns into the venous line. The venous line is then attached to the venous needle. The dialysate fluid is turned on. Gloves should be worn during this process. If the hands come into contact with patient's blood, they should immediately be washed with soap and water to avoid possible contamination with hepatitis virus.

When an *external shunt* is used, the connecting component of the shunt is removed and the Silastic® cannulae are attached to the arterial and venous lines of the dialyzer. During this process, the external portions of the shunt must be carefully protected. The operator must follow the same precautions as mentioned above.

CLOSED-CIRCUIT DIALYSIS SYSTEMS

Pl. 9

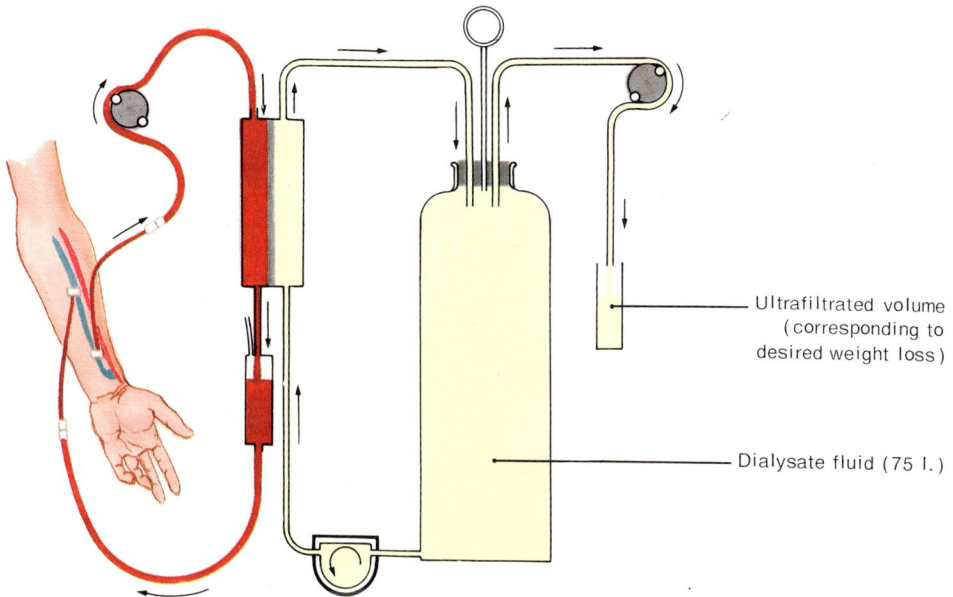

Ultrafiltrated volume (corresponding to desired weight loss)

Dialysate fluid (75 l.)

RHODIAL 75® device

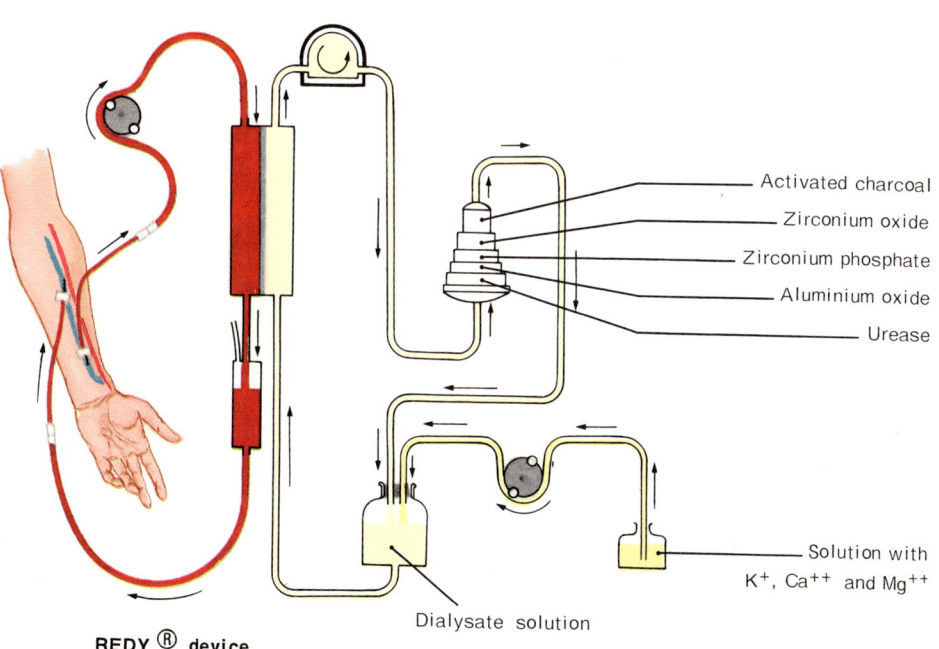

Activated charcoal
Zirconium oxide
Zirconium phosphate
Aluminium oxide
Urease

Solution with K^+, Ca^{++} and Mg^{++}

Dialysate solution

REDY® device

Single needle dialysis : when fistula puncture with two needles is difficult, a double channel needle may be used. An alternating clamp occludes the outflow line when inflow is open, and reciprocally. Partial recirculation of blood lowers dialysis efficacy, but the published reports are promising [80].

3. *Heparinization* (plate 19).

Coagulation of the extracorporeal blood, while passing through the blood lines and the dialyzer is avoided by the use of heparin.

General heparinization involves all the patient's blood, intra and extracorporeal. It is a simple system and therefore the most used. Two techniques are available. *Discontinuous* heparinization utilizes an initial 50 mg dose of sodium heparinate injected into the arterial line as soon as it is connected to the dialyzer; thereafter, 25 mg doses are injected every 2 hours. *Continuous* heparinization uses the same initial dose, but is followed by a continuous perfusion of sodium heparinate at the rate of 10 mg/hour, using a constant perfusion pump. In both systems, it is sometimes necessary to neutralize the residual heparin at the end of the dialysis session by protamine sulfate.

In local heparinization, a constant, equal dose of protamine neutralizes the heparin when it exits from the dialyzer. This technique may be necessary when there is risk of hemorrhage, for example after surgery or trauma, or during a pericarditis episode or a cerebrovascular accident. A sodium heparinate solution is continuously perfused by a constant flow pump at the rate of 15 mg/hour; simultaneous neutralization is achieved by protamine perfusion at 15 mg/hour in the venous exit from the dialyzer. One precaution is to be sure that heparin is not suddenly pulled into the arterial circuit by the blood pump.

4. *Regulation of ultrafiltration*

The desired weight loss should be decided at the beginning of the dialysis session. It should equal the difference between the pre-dialysis weight of the patient and the optimum basal weight attained at the end of the previous sessions, i.e., the weight at which the patient is normotensive. The ultrafiltration required to attain this weight should be maintained throughout the dialysis session. The method of adjusting the pressure gradient between the blood and the dialysate depends on the type of equipment. It is especially easy to regulate with Rhodial®-type equipment, where the ultrafiltrate collects in a graduated recipient.

5. *End of dialysis and blood restitution* (plate 20)

At the end of the dialysis session, the arterial needle is withdrawn and hemostasis at the puncture point is achieved by light pressure and massage. The arterial line is connected to a container of heparinized isotonic salt solution. The blood pump is stopped and the blood which remains in the dialyzer and the venous tubing is returned to the patient by gravity. The dialyzer is raised in a vertical position to the top of its stand, at about 2 meters from the floor. The blood then flows progressively back to the patient, pushed by the salt solution. Restitution by air pressure in the arterial line is not recommended since it has been responsible for massive gas embolism.

6. *Reuse of dialyzers*

Reuse of the same dialyzer for two, three or more dialyses in the same patient is of great interest economically. It can been performed manually, or with the aid of semi-automated devices which rinse and then fill the dialyzers with an antibacterial solution.

7. *Clinical surveillance of the dialysis session* (plate 21)

Clinical surveillance is necessary during each session. It mainly concerns the general state of the patient and variations in his arterial blood pressure, which should be measured and noted each hour, or more frequently if necessary. The pressure in the blood line and the negative pressure in the dialysate fluid should be noted regularly and adjusted if needed. At

MONITORING DEVICES

Pl. 10

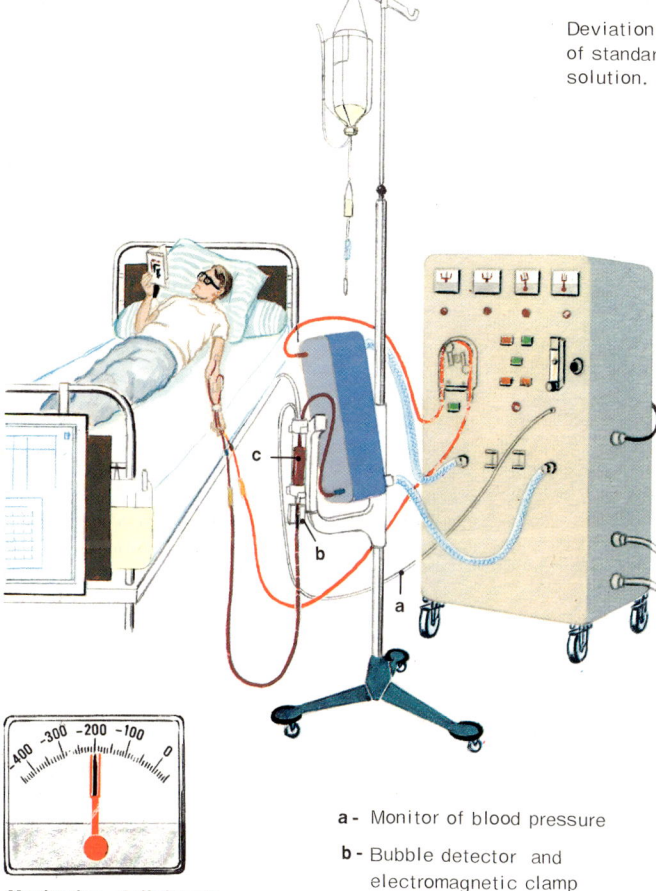

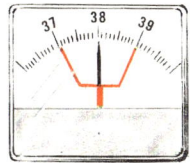

Deviation % of standard solution.

Monitoring of dialysate osmolality by conductivimeter
(alarm : ± 3.5 %)

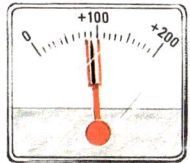

Monitoring of dialysate temperature
(alarm : ± 1° C)

a - Monitor of blood pressure
b - Bubble detector and electromagnetic clamp
c - Bubble trap

Monitoring of dialysate pressure
(alarm : ± 10 mm Hg)

Monitoring of blood line pressure at the exit from dialyzer
(alarm : ± 10 mm Hg)

Dialysate flowmeter

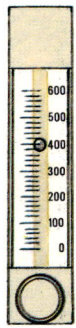

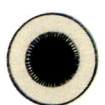

Adjustment of dialysate pressure, controlling ultrafiltration.

Adjustment of dialysate flow and dialysate pressure must be independant of each other.

the beginning and the end of the dialysis session, the blood pressure should be measured both while standing and while lying down, and the patient's weight should be measured.

All this information, noted by the nurse (or by the patient himself during home dialysis), should be recorded in a dialysis notebook or on cards for future computer analysis. Any incidents during the session should also be noted.

7.2. Incidents and accidents during the hemodialysis session

> **Incidents, and even accidents may occur during the hemodialysis session. They can almost always be avoided with strict techniques.**

They are listed below in alphabetical order:

- **Air embolism** [81]: In minor forms, this is the formation of foam in the return blood line; it may be undetected by the air detector, so that the bubble trap should be closely watched. Its severe form is due to massive entry of air after solute perfusion above the blood pump. This technique is not recommended. Emergency treatment of massive embolism is the use of a hyperbaric chamber.
- **Angor**: The occurrence of chest pain usually reflects the aggravation of pre-existing coronary insufficiency, due to reduction of circulating blood volume during the dialysis session (extra-corporeal priming volume, decrease of plasma volume by ultrafiltration). The best treatment is restoring hematocrit by blood transfusion. If compatible blood is not available, the session can be aborted and the blood in the dialyzer restored to the patient. When angor persists despite transfusion, the possibility of an acute myocardial infarction should be considered.
- **Cardiac arrhythmias** frequently occur at the end of dialysis sessions, suggesting the role of *hypokalemia*;

— sino-atrial tachycardia inconstantly accompanies blood pressure drops (see collapse, hypotension);

— tachyarrhythmia can appear at the end of a dialysis session, when blood potassium is at its lowest. ECG tracing will indicate the type of disorder. It is usually a variable type of extrasystolic tachyarrhythmia, sometimes with atrial fibrillation or flutter. These arrhythmias often reflect *latent coronary insufficiency.* They can be prevented or improved by using a dialysate enriched for potassium ions. They generally disappear after potassium ingestion, or after blood transfusion in anemic patients.

- **Chest pain** have two main causes:

— Angor (see that term)
— Pericarditis: chest pain during dialysis should always lead to the search of pericardial friction rub.

- **Chills** are often associated with fever and have the same three possible causes (see fever). They may also be due to a low temperature of the dialysate fluid or to acute hemolysis resulting from a hypoosmotic dialysate (see hemolysis).
- **Coagulation in the blood circuit** can take any of three aspects:

— massive coagulation, making blood restitution impossible and thus increasing anemia. In each case, the decision must be made whether to transfuse the patient or to re-initiate the dialysis with a new dialyzer;

WATER TREATEMENT FOR DIALYSIS

Pl. 11

Schematic representation of an ideal set-up

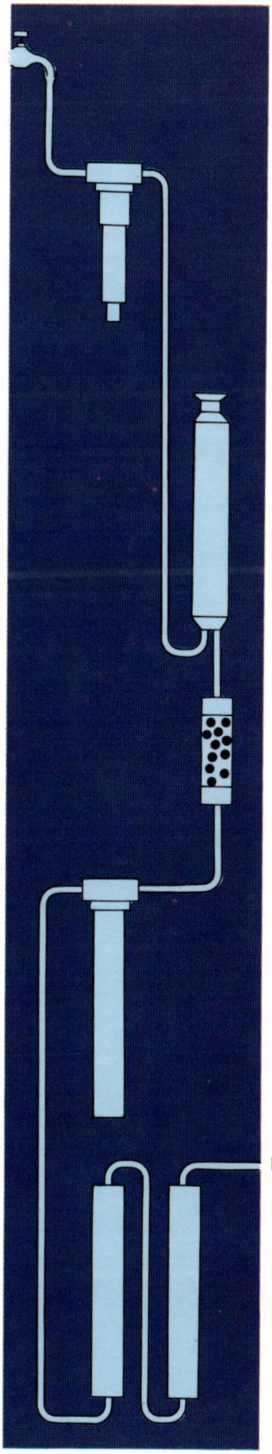

Tap water

Device:	Successive removing of:
Sedimentation filter	Particles larger than 5 microns
Water softener	Calcium Magnesium (+ release of sodiums ions)
Charcoal filters	Chloramines Organic substances Pyrogens
Reverse osmosis	About 90% of solutes

Highly purified water ($\geqslant 0{,}3\ M\Omega/cm^2$)

Deionizer	Sodium Carbonate, sulfate, chloride, nitrate Fe, Mn, Al

Tardieu

— partial coagulation, restricted to a few circuits of a parallel plate dialyzer, results only in diminishing the efficiency of dialysis, which usually can be continued ;

— repeated coagulations suggest such factors as elevated hematocrit, low blood flow or a spontaneous tendency to clot. In patients who have unexplained tendency to thrombosis, the use of platelet anti-aggregants and/or dicoumarinics may be useful.

● **Convulsions** : convulsions usually have a vascular or metabolic origin, such as :

— *hypertension* complicated by cerebral edema (see headaches) : this mostly occures in patients whose basic blood pressure levels are poorly controlled ;

— *cerebro-vascular accident* : this accident is most often induced by arterial hypertension and favored by chronic anticoagulant treatment or by heparinization used during dialysis ;

— *hypercalcemia,* as part of the hard-water syndrome (see that term) ;

— *severe hypocalcemia* associated with too rapid correction of acidosis, observed principally during first hemodialysis sessions or after vomiting ;

— *preexisting comitiality :* initiate or adjust treatment.

Emergency treatment of grand mal seizures includes i.m. or i.v. administration of Diazépam (Valium®), needing possibly ventilatory assistance, or i.v. infusion of Clometiazole.

● **Cramps** : Contrary to an earlier opinion, cramps almost never result from hypocalcemia but are almost always due to *sodium depletion.* When cramps occur during each dialysis session despite adequate ultrafiltration, the dialysate sodium concentration should be raised, e.g. to about 145 mEq/l, if a dialysis fluid with lower sodium concentration was previously used. Cramps can also reflect uremic *polyneuritis,* either evolving or regressing. They can sometimes be calmed by high doses of vitamin B_6 or by quinine derivatives.

● **Electrical breakdown** : it brings stoppage of the blood pump, the heating apparatus, circulation of the dialysate fluid and all monitoring devices. Action to be taken depends on the length of the breakdown :

— if it is *less than 30 seconds,* no serious incident can occur ;

— if it lasts *longer than 30 seconds,* the blood pump should be kept turning by hand (if the apparatus is so equipped). If, not, the blood line should be removed from the pump and the blood circuit left to move by arterial pressure ; an additional dose of heparin should be injected. It is often useful to compress the fistula lightly between the arterial and venous needless to reduce return pressure. It is possible to maintain blood circulation in this manner for about 15 minutes without coagulation ;

— if the breakdown lasts *more than 15 minutes,* the dialysis session should be interrumpted and the blood returned.

● **Fever** : Three possible causes should be distinguished :

— transient fever, with negative blood cultures which spontaneously disappears a few hours after the dialysis session is usually due to passage of bacterial endotoxins from the dialysate fluid to the blood ;

— persistent fever, continuing after the end of the session, with positive blood cultures, often reflects infection of vascular access and should be carefully watched ;

— more rarely, fever during a dialysis session can be due to an intolerance for blood or protamine infusion.

● **Hard water syndrome** is a syndrome related to acute hypercalcemia, up to or above 14 mg/100 ml, occurring during a hemodialysis session, and due to an excessive concentration of calcium in the dialysate fluid [44]. It can result from the use of « hard » water, i.e. water containing more than 8 mg/100 ml calcium. In practice, it is usually seen when the water

HEMOFILTRATION

Pl. 12

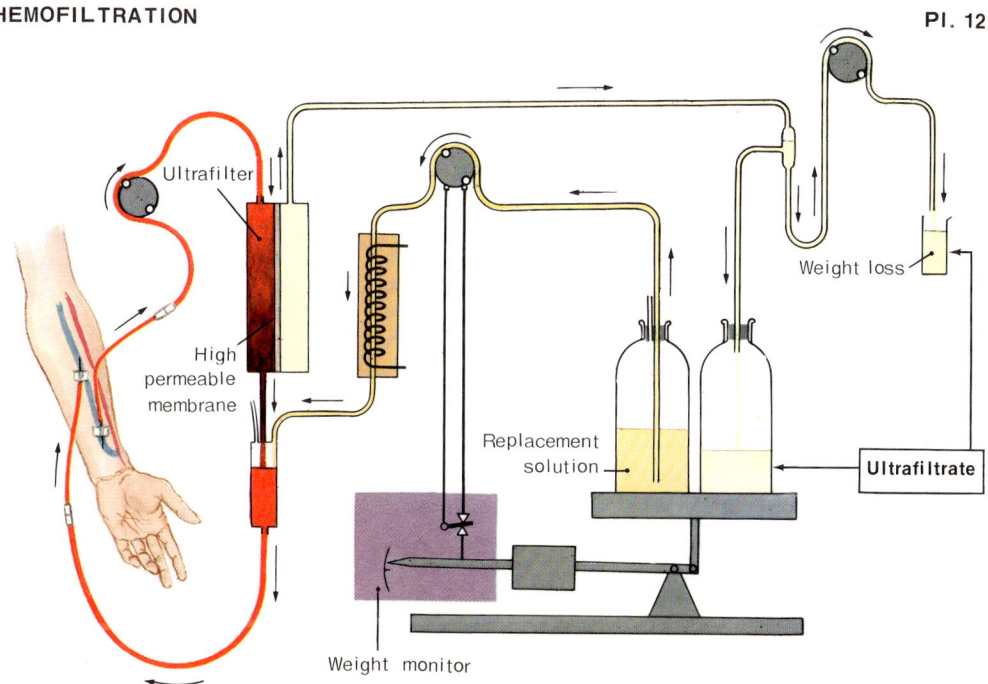

Hemofiltration device using post-dilution

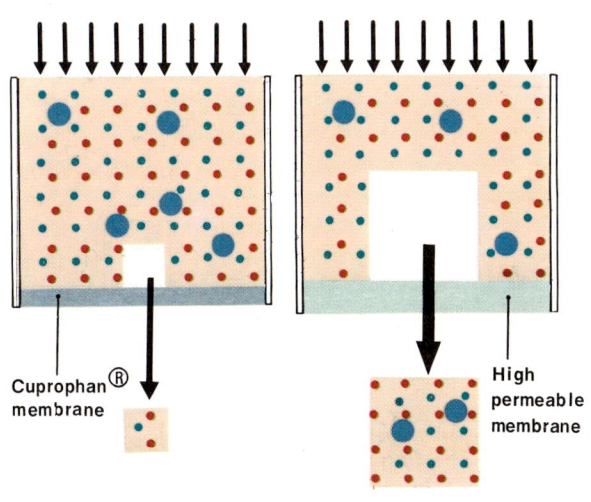

For a given hydrostatic pressure and membrane surface area, the volume of solvent and the amount of solutes transfered are greater with high permeable membranes than with Cuprophan®. Moreover, the former only allows substantial transfer of "middle molecules".

Principles of hemofiltration

softener resins are worn out. Clinical manifestations are headache, nausea, vomiting, sometimes « red eyes », increased blood pressure and then convulsions.

The disorder is reversible with the return to normal levels of calcium.

- **Headaches :** there are three main causes of headache during dialysis :

— *hypertensive reaction* to rapid water and sodium depletion due to ultrafiltration, possibly via renin-angiotensin stimulation or by liberation of catecholamines. Treatment consists of stopping or reducing ultrafiltration. Sometimes, it can be due to an excessive reduction of plama volume resulting from a hyperosmotic dialysate. In this case, the bath concentration must be rapidly adjusted ;

— *hypercalcemia* secondary to the use of water which is too rich in calcium (see « hard water » syndrome) ;

— *hemolysis* due to hypo-osmotic dialysate fluid (see hemolysis).

Intense headache may be observed in the absence of any of the above causes. Sometimes an excessive pressure in the venous network seems to be responsible.

- **Hematoma :**

— *A superficial hematoma* around the puncture point is usually due to unsuccessful insertion of a needle. Sometimes, the dialysis session will have to be interrupted and the following session postponed. Surgical drainage will be necessary if the hematoma is compressive and threatens thrombosis of the fistula or if it is extensive, taking excessive blood.

— *A deep hematoma* can occur because of heparinization, after biopsy or surgery. The following dialysis should then be postponed for a minimum of 36 to 48 hours and should be performed with local heparinization.

- **Hemolysis (acute) :** serious but rare complication, acute hemolysis is almost always caused by osmotic imbalance in the blood following an error in composition of the dialysate fluid, undetected by the conductivity monitor. First signs are blood pressure drop, oppression, nausea, hedache, then convulsions and coma. The blood is a lacquer red, but this may be hidden by the thickness of the tubing. Usually, hemolysis results from *excessive dilution* or omission of the concentrate. Rapid diagnosis can be made if the bath does not taste salty and by testing the bath with a *portable conductivity monitor* (this apparatus should be available in every center) and by measuring dialysate sodium concentration. Also, hemolysis can result from *hypernatremia.* due to water softener malfunction [82]. Rarely, hemolysis can be due to *overheating* of the dialysate fluid [83] or to *traces of formaline* (or

Treatment is immediate interruption of the dialysis session and re-initiation after correction of the dialysate composition. In severe cases, immediate exchange transfusion is necessary. It can be made with preserved blood, with the citrate and potassium being eliminated by the dialysis.

- **Hypertension :** a hypertensive episode during dialysis usually results from too rapid ultrafiltration in a patient who is hypertensive between dialyses. It is manifested by headache and possibly convulsions (see those two words).

- **Hypotension :**

— *progressive hypotension* usually reflects an effect of ultrafiltration. It is particularly seen in normotensive, anephric patients. However, sometimes the blood pressure drop due to ultrafiltration occurs suddenly. It is inconstantly associated with tachycardia and *orthostatic hypotension,* which can persist several hours after the end of the dialysis session. It can usually be avoided by precluding the necessity for high ultrafiltration, i.e. by limiting the weight gain between dialyses. When excessive interdialytic weight gain does not seem to be the factor responsible, the basal weight of the patient should be reevaluated. Immediate

PERFORMANCE OF DIALYZERS

Pl. 13

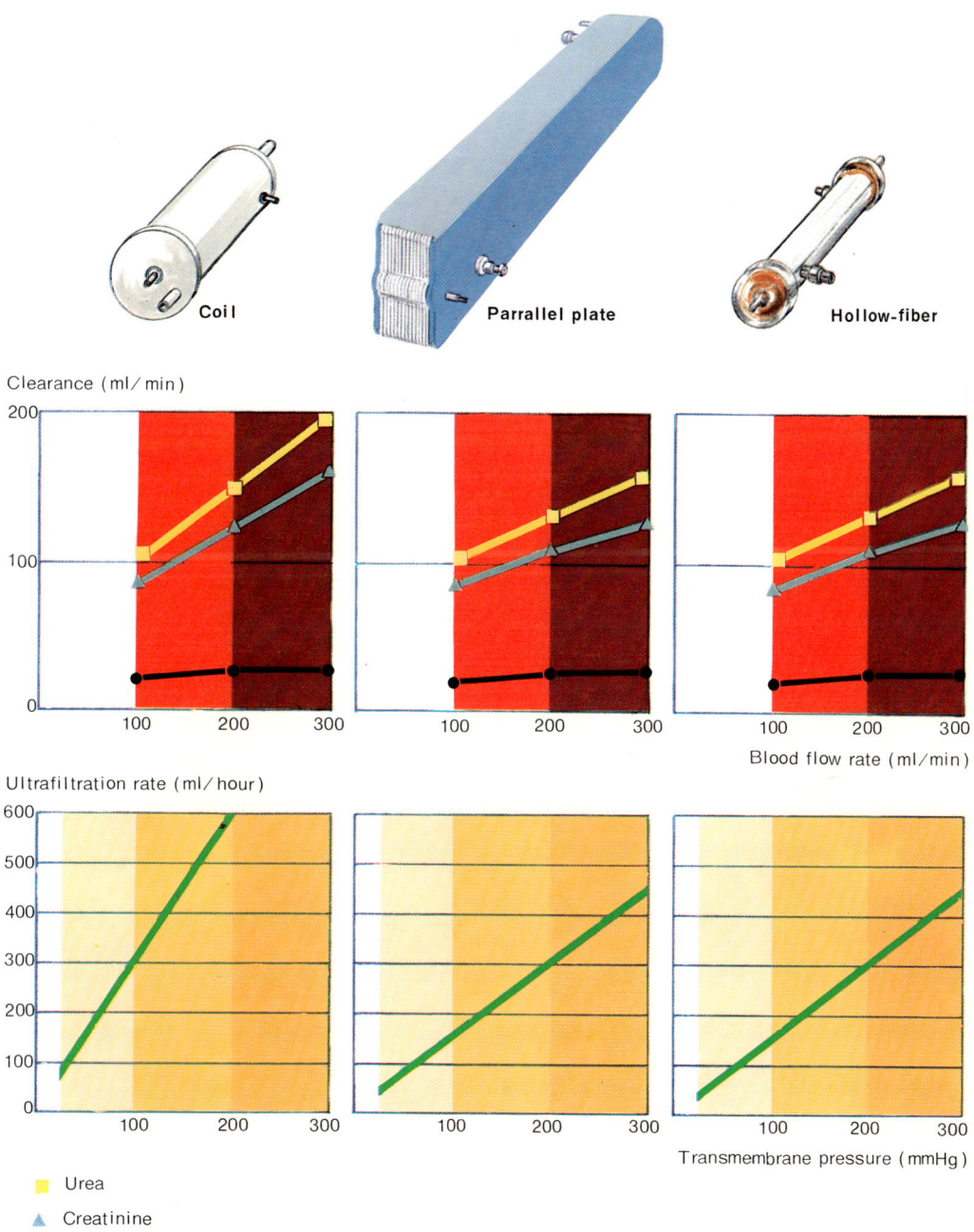

■ Urea
▲ Creatinine
● Vitamin B12

Mean clearance and ultrafiltration rates of dialyzers using 1 m² Cuprophan® membranes
(Hemodialysis laboratory, Necker Hospital)

treatment should be lowering the patient's head, perfusing isotonic saline and stopping ultrafiltration;

— *rapid blood pressure drop* during dialysis, associated with manifestations of acute right ventricular insufficiency (painful hepatomegaly, swollen jugular veins) suggests acute pericardial tamponade induced by heparinization. When it is associated with stenocardiac pain, a myocardial infarction must be considered (see precordialgias);

— some *hypotensive drugs* (alphamethyldopa, guanethidine) induce rapid blood pressure drop during water and sodium depletion;

— lastly, hypotension may signal internal or external *hemorrhage,* such as membrane rupture or accidental or voluntary removal of needles or cannulae (see collapse).

• **Membrane rupture**: because of the pressure regimens in blood and dialysate circuits, membrane rupture causes blood to flow into the dialysate fluid. Ideally, it should be detected immediately; in practice, its detection varies with the equipment used;

— if the dialysis bath is visible, a pink or red color indicates membrane rupture;

— if the dialysis bath is not visible, a monitoring device should detect any blood leakage and stop the bloop pump.

However, a certain quantity of blood will continue to be pulled into the dialysis bath because of its negative pressure. Aeterial and venous lines should thus be clamped and the session interrupted, or re-initiated with a new dialyzer if the accident occurred near the beginning of the dialysis.

• **Menorrhage**: Functionnal menorrhagia, secondary to the lutein deficiency often seen in hemodialyzed women, increase during dialyses performed during the menstrual period. It is improved by luteinizing hormone treatment. As with metrorragia, gynecological examination should seek an associated organic disorder.

• **Nausea**: see vomiting.

• **Precordialgias**: they have two principal causes:

— *coronary insufficiency*: precordialgia is often induced by hypovolemia, due to the weight loss produced by ultrafiltration, and by anemia (see angor). An ECG is required to eliminate the possibility of myocardial infarction, when precordialgia persists despite transfusion of red blood cells;

— *pericarditis*: the pain can be similar to that of angina. It is generally increased by dorsal decubitus and relieved by the sitting position. Diagnosis is confirmed by detection of pericardial friction rub and by chest X-ray and echocardiography. Sudden hypotension, with or without signs of right ventricular failure, may indicate acute hemopericardium with tamponade.

• **Pruritus**: it appears due to the presence of microscopic deposits of calcium phosphate in the skin when the phosphocalcic product exceeds 75. It can be aggravated during dialysis sessions because the increase in plasma calcium is more rapid than the decrease in plasma phosphate. The best long-term treatment is decreasing plasma phosphate concentration.

• **Pulmonary edema** (acute): a frequent emergency situation in dialyzed patients, is usually due to water and sodium overload between dialysis. In some cases pulmonary edema reflects pericarditis, pre-existing valvular disease or uremic cardiomyopathy.

When it appears during a dialysis session, myocardial infarction or pulmonary embolism is suggested.

Emergency treatment of pulmonary edema resulting from water and sodium overload is immediate dialysis with rapid ultrafiltration. The most useful dialysis membranes for this purpose are those with high hydraulic permeability. When the edema occurs outside the

MAIN TYPES OF VASCULAR ACCESS

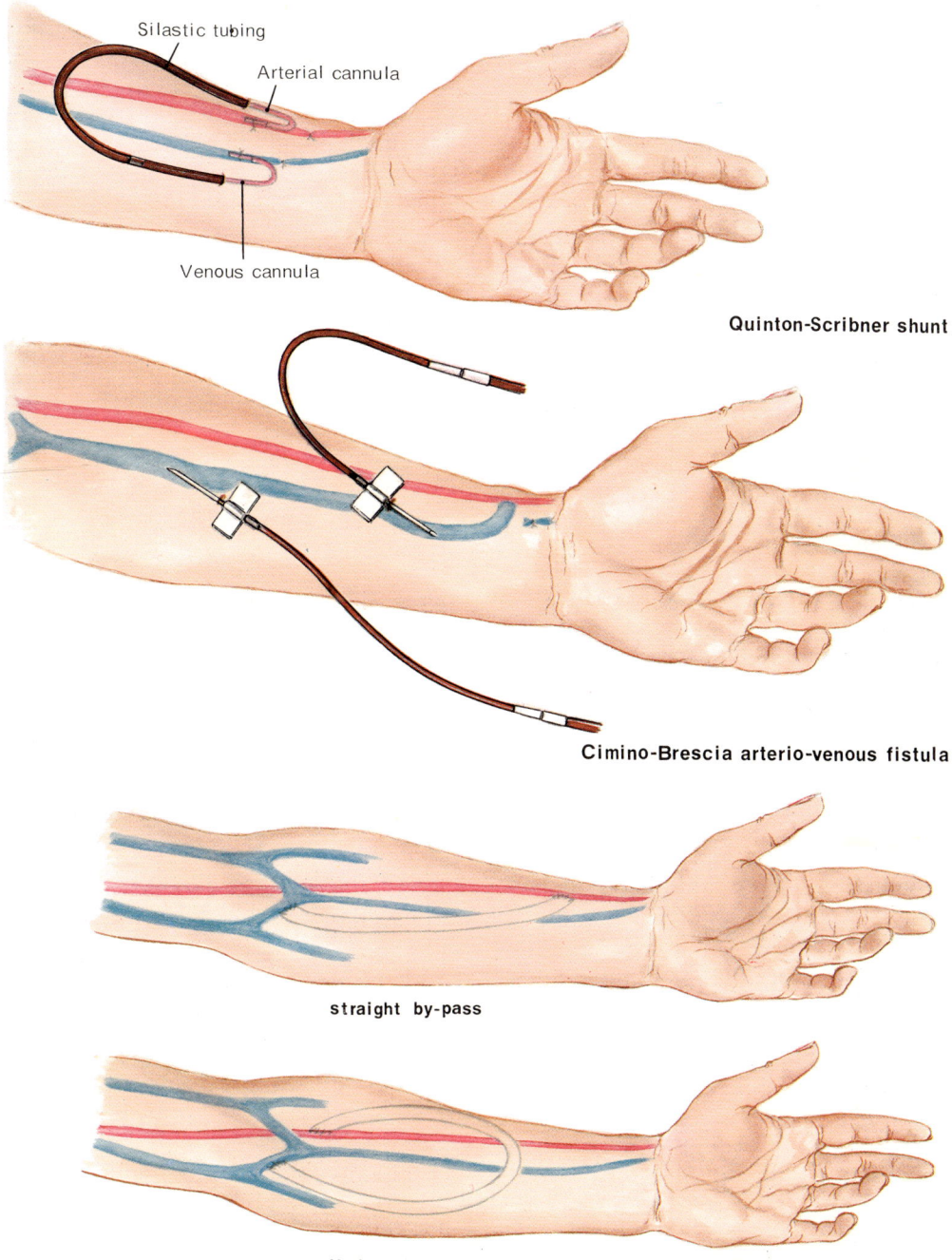

dialysis center, treatment should be lowering of arterial hypertension by rapidly-effective hypotensive drugs such as Diazoxide administered intravenously or Clonidine (Catapressan®), administered intramuscularly, associated with Furosemid injection (Lasilix®) intravenously. In cases of extreme emergency, bleeding may be necessary : this can only be considered if the patient's hematocrit is not too low.

- **Puncture point bleeding** : Bleeding can occur around the puncture points when the fistula or the arteriovenous graft lacks elasticity. If it occurs during dialysis, hemostatic adhesive gauze (Surgical®) should be placed around the points.

If it occurs after the needles are withdrawn, light pressure should be applied, while « massaging » the puncture point, taking care not to compress the fistula.

- **Vascular collapse** should suggest the search for :

— too rapid extracellular *fluid volume depletion* leading to hypotension : ultrafiltration should be stopped or decreased ;

— undetected *bleeding :* watch for the appearance of a melaena ;

— undetected *membrane rupture* in the dialyzer : check the color of the lines and whether the alarms are functioning properly.

- **Vomiting** (or nausea) occurs frequently during dialysis. It has various significations :

— during the first dialyses, it generally reflects *osmotic imbalance* and can be avoided by progressively increasing the number of hours of dialysis ;

— associated with headaches, it often reflects an *increase in blood pressure* (see headache) ;

— associated with headache and often a rapid increase in blood pressure, it can manifest a « *hard water syndrome* » (see that term) ;

— associated with blood pressure drop and headache, it can indicate *acute hemolysis* (see that term) ;

— vomiting can sometimes occur which is not associated with any of these mechanisms. When *associated with abdominal pain,* it favors diagnoses such as hepatitis, pancreatitis, gastroduodenal ulcer, cholelithiasis, or infection of a polycystic or lithiasic kidney.

7.3. Clinical and biochemical control of the hemodialysis patient

> Controls include laboratory examinations at regular intervals and complete clinical examination at least four times a year.

7.3.1. Laboratory follow-up

Regular laboratory examinations are necessary to determine dialysis efficacy. They should be kept to a minimum to avoid drawing unnecessary blood. Examinations are made predialysis, usually once a week or every two weeks or even monthly in stable home dialysis patients. A post-dialysis analysis is less frequently necessary.

Blood levels of the following parameters are usually determined :

— urea, creatinine, uric acid, total protein, hematocrit,
— sodium, potassium, chloride, bicarbonate, calcium, phosphate.

HEMODIALYSIS EQUIPMENT

Pl. 15

1- Dakin solution
2- Material for fistula puncture
   (compress, gloves, tourniquet, adhesive strips)
3- Alcohol
4- Heparin
5- Needles
6- Heparin syringe
7- Venous line
8- Clamps
9- Sterile towels
10- Heparin and protamin pump
11- Bubble trap
12- Dialyzer
13- Arterial line
14- Normal saline
15- Dialysate concentration monitor dial
    (conductivimeter)
16- Dialysate temperature monitor dial
17- Blood pressure monitor dial
18- Dialysate pressure monitor dial
19- Dialysate flowmeter
20- Blood pump
21- Dialysate line

a- Stop
b- Start
c- Dialysis
d- Sterilisation
e- Preparation
f- Pump

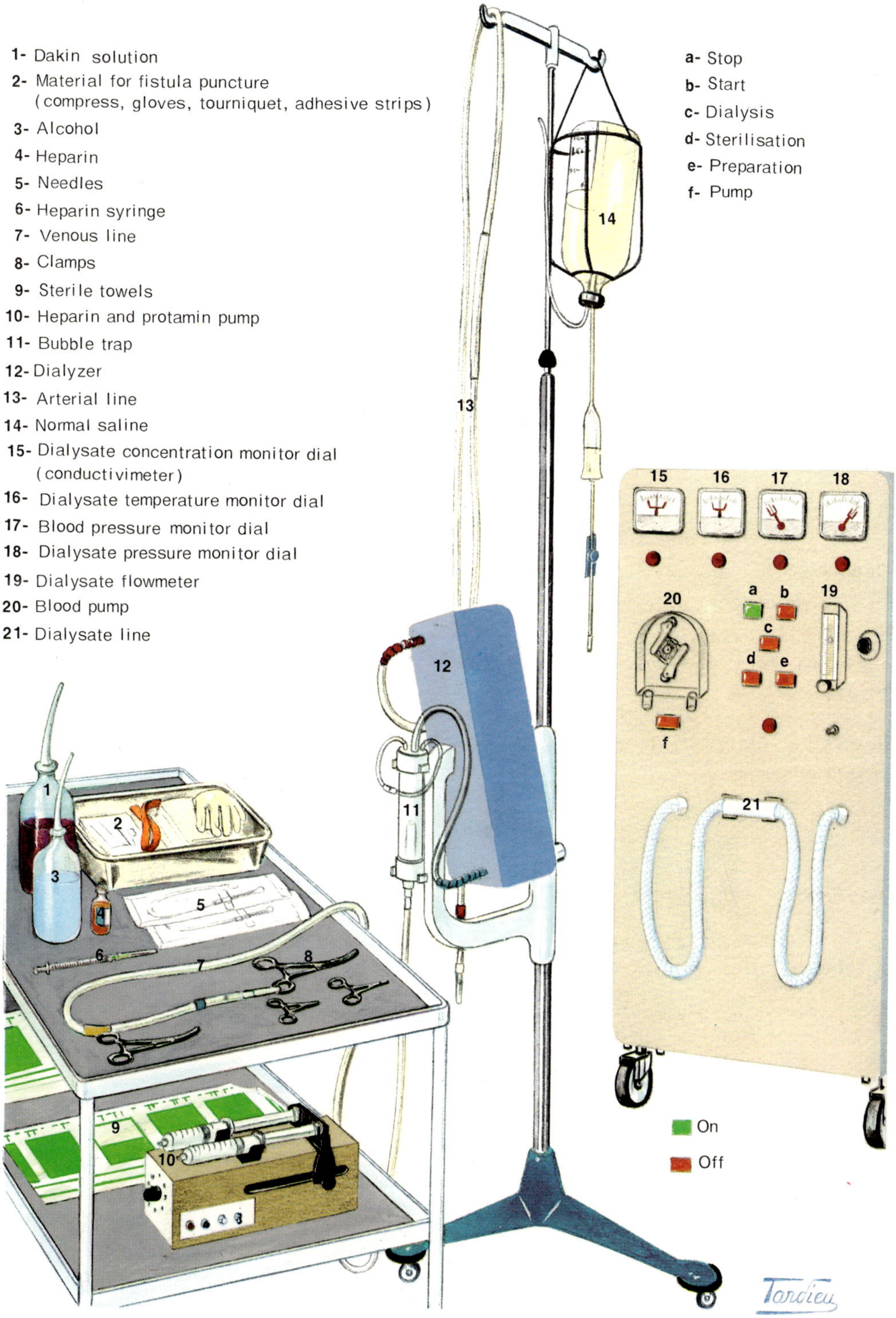

On
Off

These data may be fed into a computer, which can then furnish mean monthly data for each patient.

Pre-dialysis plasma levels of urea and creatinine indicate dialysis efficiency with regard to light molecular weight solutes, as well as the nutritional status of the patient. Mean values before and after dialysis, for three sessions per week on a 1 m² Cuprophan® membrane, are shown in the table below (table II, p. 63).

When blood urea is inappropriately low when compared with blood creatinine, protein intake may be insufficient. Conversely, when creatinine concentration is proportionally lower than urea concentration, a decrease in muscular mass or excessive protein intake is suggested.

There are as yet no routine criteria for determining « middle molecule » removal.

At the present time, clinical examination provides the best long-term assessment of dialysis adequacy.

7.3.2. Long-term clinical follow-up

Clinical examination, performed routinely every three months, should particularly aim at the following points:

1. *Overall results* of dialysis: general status, psychological adaptation, what physical activity is possible for the patient.

2. *Nutritional state:* observance of diet and water restrictions; mean weight gain between dialyses. Estimation of daily protein intake. Residual diuresis, noting intercurrent nephrectomy which may have led to the anephric state. Serum level of lipids, cholesterol, and triglycerides; electrophoresis of serum proteins.

3. *Vascular access:* thrombosis or infection; blood flow rate; cardiac tolerance of the arteriovenous fistula.

4. *Solute removal and electrolyte balance;* mean predialysis plasma concentrations of urea, creatinine, uric acid, sodium, potassium and bicarbonate.

5. *Cardiovascular* examination: control of hypertension and possible requirement of hypotensive drugs; search for congestive heart failure, pericardial friction rub, angor, cardiac arrhythmias, chest X-rays, ECG and optic fundi.

6. *Neurological* examination: clinical manifestations of uremic polyneuritis; motor-nerve conduction velocity (MNCV) at the common peroneal nerve.

7. *Gastrointestinal* examination: existence of virus B hepatitis, follow-up of course by HBs antigen detection and corresponding antibody; determination of serum transaminases, alkaline phosphatases, bilirubin. Determination of serum immunoglobulins and BSP clearance in the case of chronic heptitis. G-I barium enema if indicated.

8. Analysis of *calcium and phosphorus metabolism:* pruritus, bone pain, plasma concentrations of calcium and phosphorus before and after dyalysis. Determination of serum alkaline phosphatase. X-rays of hands and pelvis. If necessary, assessment of plasma parathyroid hormone level and plasma concentration of vitamin D metabolites, or bone biopsy.

9. *Hematological* examinations: tolerance of anemia, transfusions required, hematocrit, hemoglobin, plasma iron and iron binding capacity; assessment of RBC, leukocyte (including differential leukocyte count), platelet and reticulocyte count.

10. *Overall evaluation of dialysis*: general state, psychological tolerance of treatment, professional and family activity, quality of life of the patient.

Below are summarized **complementary examinations** which should be performed every three months in all dialysis patients (in parentheses, if particularly indicated):

Serum protein and electrophoresis (determination of serum complement).

Detection of HBs antigen and anti-HBs antibody.

Serum lipids, cholesterol, triglycerides.

Serum transaminases, alkaline phosphatases, bilirubin, (BSP clearance, determination of IgG if chronic hepatitis is suspected).

Red blood cell count, hematocrit, hemoglobin, leukocyte count (with differential leukocyte count), platelets and reticulocyte count.

Serum iron, iron binding capacity.

Bacteriologic examination of urine.

Electrocardiogram.

Optic fundi.

Electromyogram. Measurement of motor-nerve conduction velocity. Radiographic examination of the thorax, the hands and the pelvis (if necessary, other bones including the skull).

Cross-match against HLA leukocyte and platelet antigens (regularly performed two weeks after any transfusion).

TABLE II

Mean predialysis plasma concentration of urea and creatinine in 1 065 chronic dialysis patients (after Degoulet et al., 1977 [6]).

Concentrations (mean + 1 SD)	Male (N = 620)	Female (N = 445)
Urea (mg/100 ml)	192 ± 39	188 ± 36
Creatinine (mg/100 ml)	13.8 ± 3.0	9.9 ± 5.0

PREPARATION OF DIALYSIS EQUIPMENT

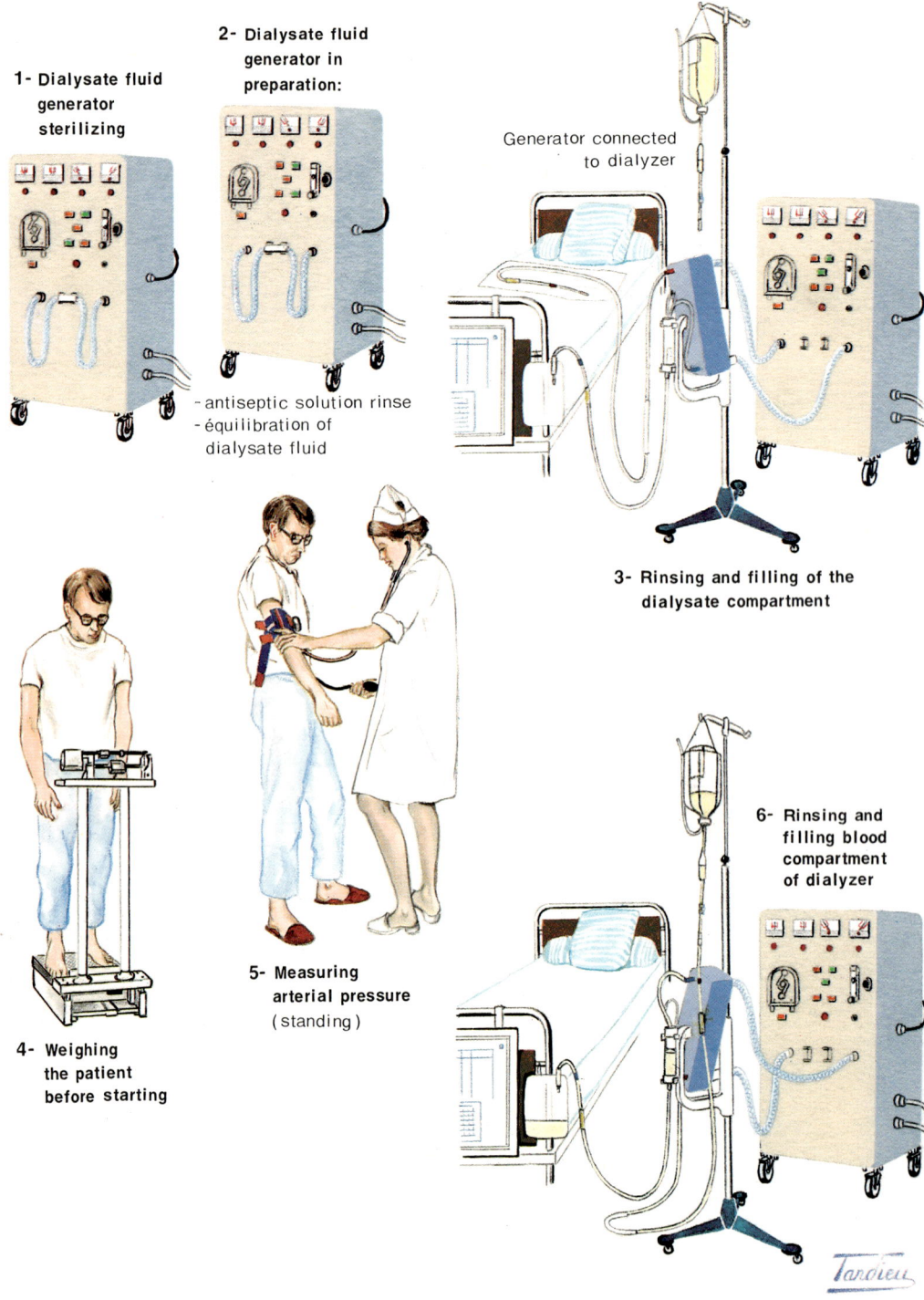

1- Dialysate fluid generator sterilizing

2- Dialysate fluid generator in preparation:
- antiseptic solution rinse
- équilibration of dialysate fluid

Generator connected to dialyzer

3- Rinsing and filling of the dialysate compartment

4- Weighing the patient before starting

5- Measuring arterial pressure (standing)

6- Rinsing and filling blood compartment of dialyzer

STARTING DIALYSIS SESSION

Pl. 17

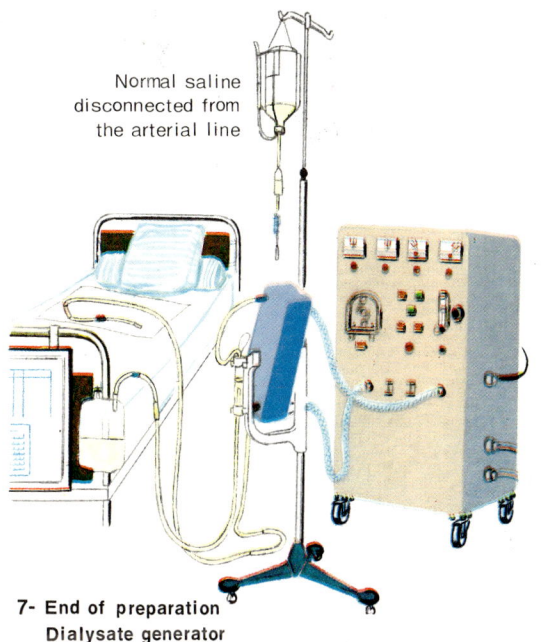

Normal saline disconnected from the arterial line

7- **End of preparation**
Dialysate generator and dialyzer ready for use

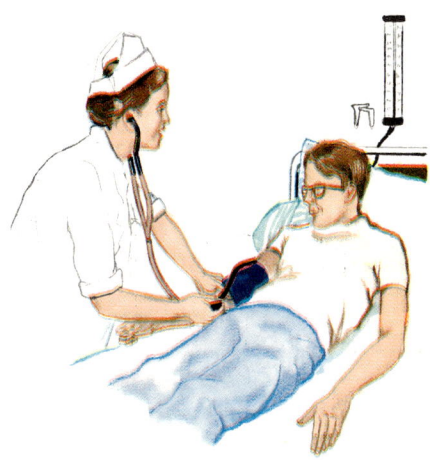

8- **Measuring blood pressure**
(supine)

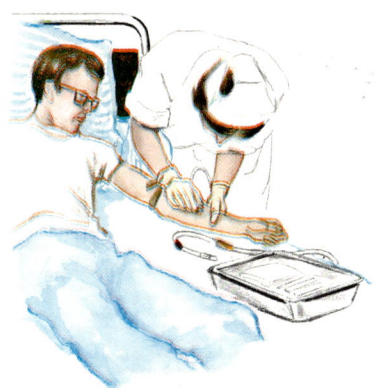

9- **Puncture of arterio-venous fistula**
Insertion of "arterial" needle

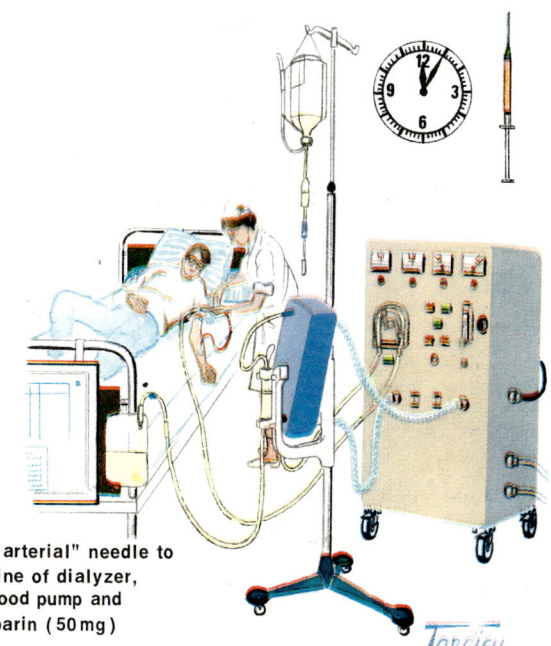

10- **Connection of the "arterial" needle to the arterial blood line of dialyzer, then start of the blood pump and priming dose of heparin (50 mg)**

VASCULAR CONNECTION

Pl. 18

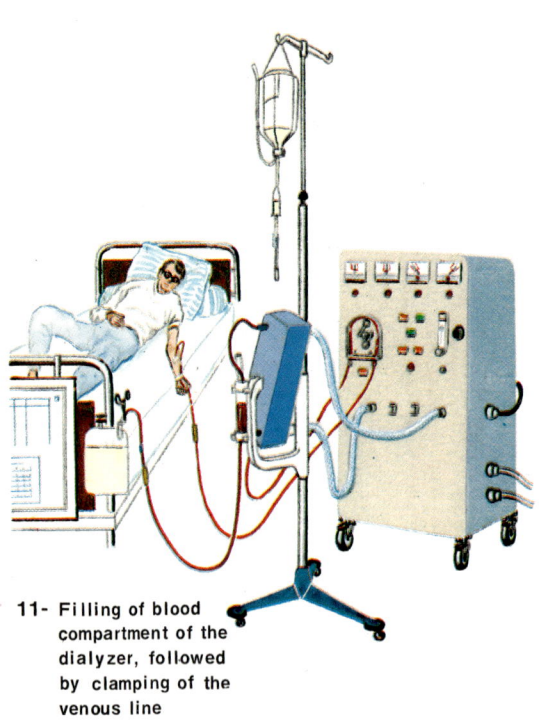

11- Filling of blood compartment of the dialyzer, followed by clamping of the venous line

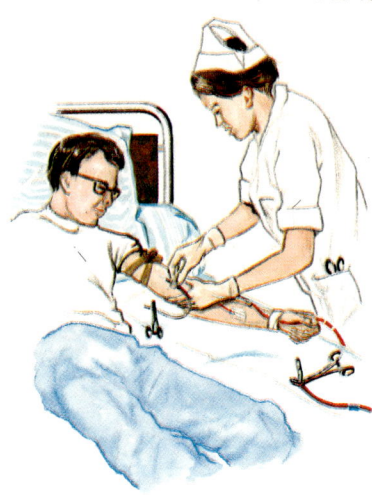

12- Insertion of the "venous" needle

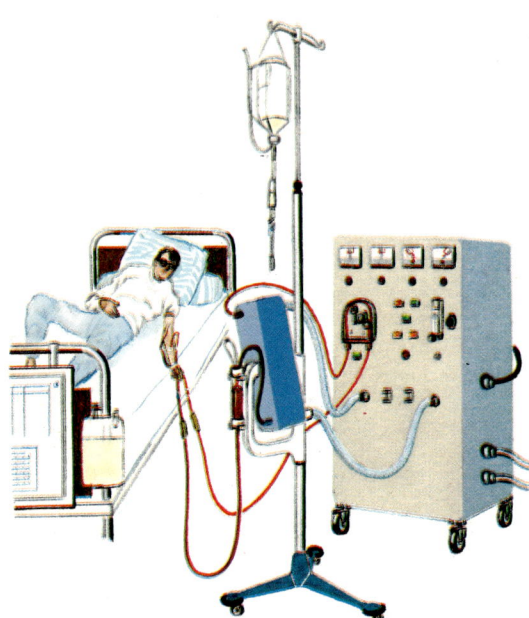

13- Connection of the "venous" needle to the venous blood line of the dialyzer

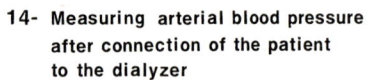

14- Measuring arterial blood pressure after connection of the patient to the dialyzer

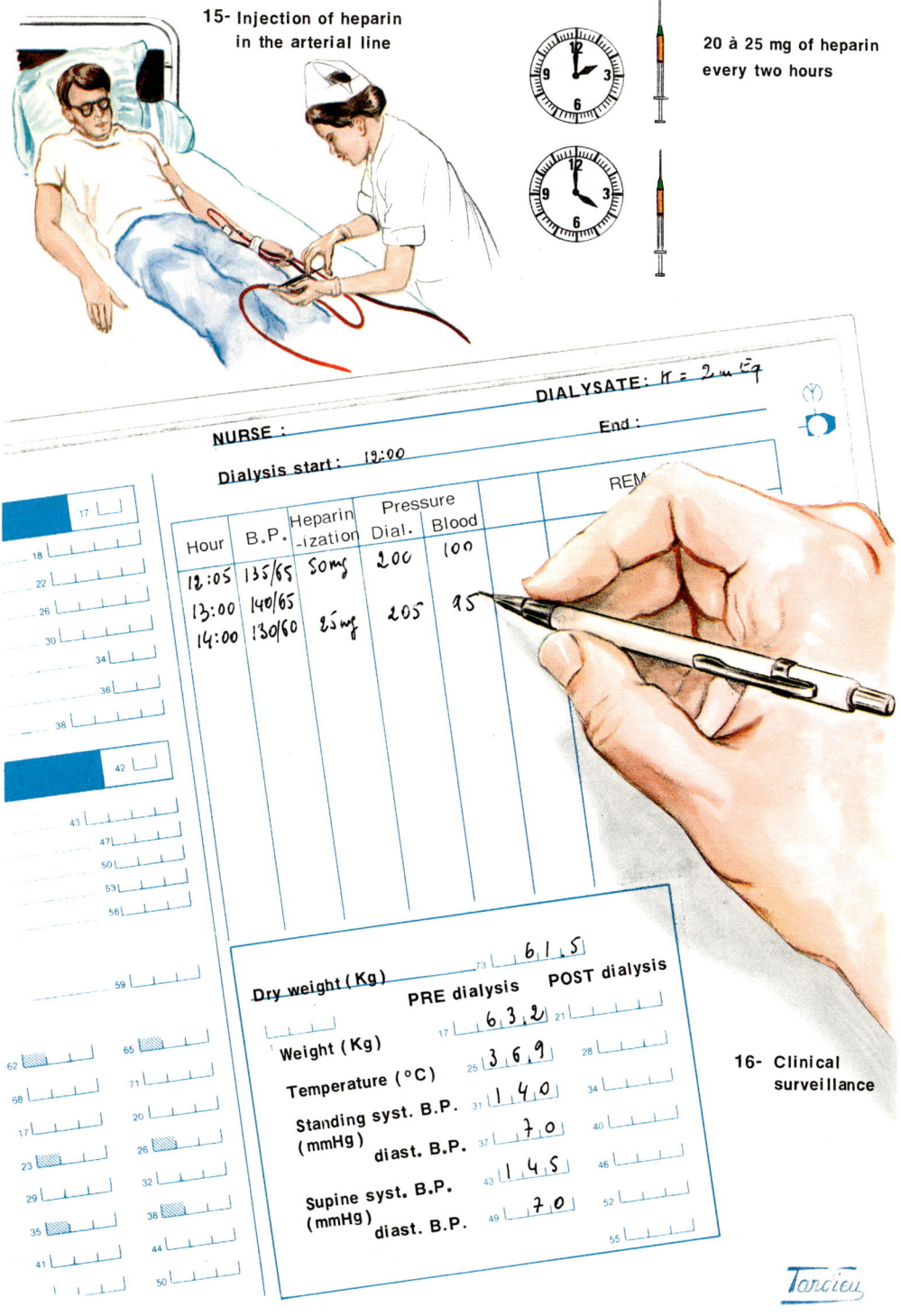

END OF DIALYSIS AND BLOOD RESTITUTION

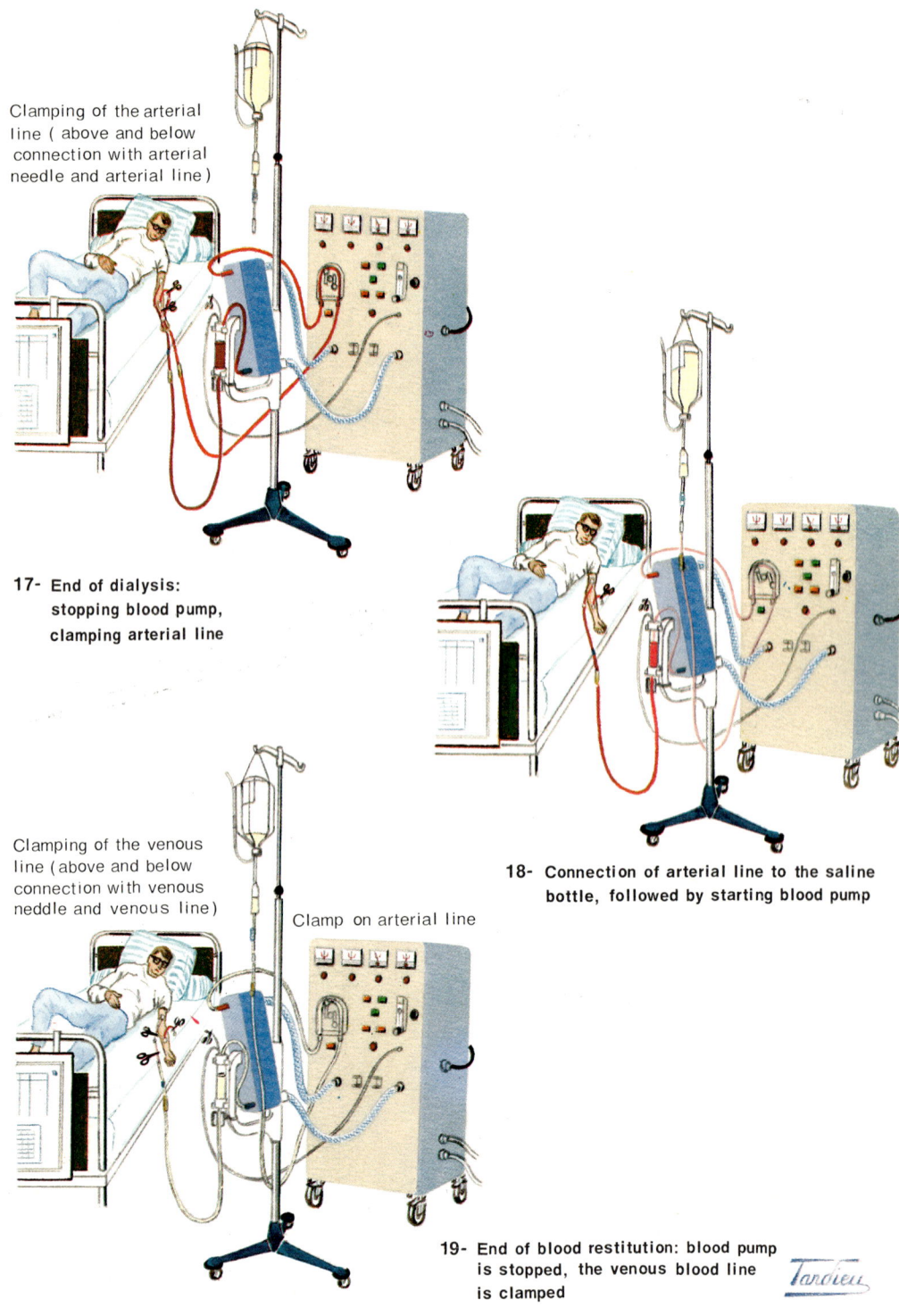

Clamping of the arterial line (above and below connection with arterial needle and arterial line)

17- End of dialysis: stopping blood pump, clamping arterial line

18- Connection of arterial line to the saline bottle, followed by starting blood pump

Clamping of the venous line (above and below connection with venous neddle and venous line)

Clamp on arterial line

19- End of blood restitution: blood pump is stopped, the venous blood line is clamped

CONTROLS AT THE END OF DIALYSIS

Pl. 21

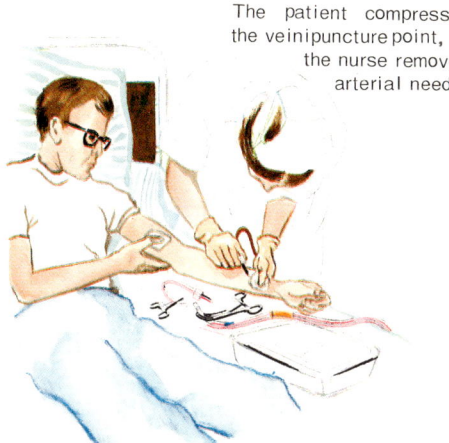

The patient compresses the veinipuncture point, as the nurse removes arterial needle

20- Compression of the venous puncture point and removal of the arterial needle

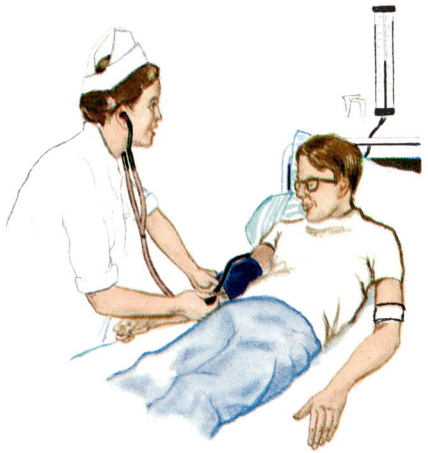

21- Measuring arterial blood pressure after disconnection from the dialyzer
(supine)

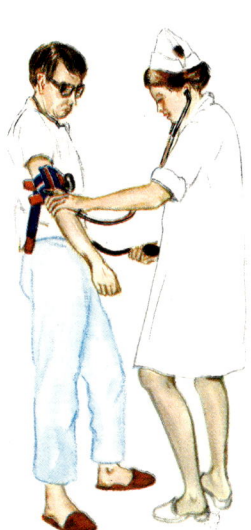

22- Measuring arterial blood pressure
(standing)

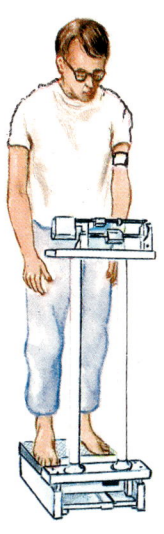

23- Weighing the patient at the end of dialysis
(control of weight loss)

VIII. CLINICAL PROBLEMS
IN CHRONIC HEMODIALYSIS PATIENTS

Visceral and metabolic complications can persist or appear during chronic hemodialysis (pl. 22).

They are due to the fact that the removal of toxic metabolites by dialysis is not as effective as that performed by normal kidneys and that endocrine and metabolic deficiencies cannot be palliated by hemodialysis. In addition, lack of adherence to dietary restrictions can produce some water and electrolyte disorders.

Much progress has been made in understanding these disorders during the last ten years. Treatment and even prevention is now possible. Thus we see a reduction in the frequency and severity of arterial hypertension, polyneuritis, renal osteodystrophy and even pericarditis in these patients. Conversely, the frequency of cardiac and cerebral atherosclerotic complications has increased with the greater mean age and longevity of patients treated by hemodialysis.

8.1. Cardiovascular problems

These problems concern mainly hypertension, arterial atherosclerosis, and cardiac disorders.

8.1.1. Arterial hypertension

Hypertension, defined by diastolic blood pressure above or equal to 9.5 mmHg is seen in about 75 percent or uremic patients at the beginning of dialysis treatment.

In most cases, it disappears with water and sodium removal by hemodialysis. It can thus be considered « *volume dependent* » [85]. In our series, nearly 60 percent of formerly hypertensive patients became normotensive during the first six months of treatment, after a volume depletion reaching 5 to 10 percent of initial body weight [86]. However, in some cases this normalization was obtained without appreciable decrease in body weight. Patients who where initially normotensive usually remained so.

In approximately 40 percent of initially hypertensive subjects, hypertension was only partially controlled by hemodialysis alone but responded to hypotensive drugs.

In about 5 percent of chronic hemodialysis patients (who nearly all suffer from vascular kidney diseases such as renal arteriosclerosis or thrombotic microangiopathy), hypertension persisted despite reducing body weight and the administration of hypotensive drugs. Such « uncontrollable » hypertension is generally associated with high renin secretion, (i.e., « *renin dependent* » hypertension), increased peripheral resistance and low cardiac output [87].

In rare cases, *bilateral nephrectomy* is necessary to control excessive renin secretion and to correct hypertension. However, binephrectomy aggravates anemia. Today, persistent hypertension can almost always be corrected medically by the use of hypotensive agents including beta-blockers which reduce the secretion of renin (propranolol or Avlocardyl®). However, some beta-blockers such as pindolol (Visken®), which do not reduce renin secretion, are also effective. Beta-blockers must frequently be associated with Hydralazine (Nepressol®), alphamethyldopa (Aldomet®) or clonidine (Catapressan®). As a result, cases in which bilateral nephrectomy is indicated are now very rare [85].

8.1.2. Vascular atherosclerosis

Diffuse atheroma, involving particularly coronary and cerebral arteries, as well as arteries of the lower limbs, is seen more frequently in uremic patients, whether dialyzed or not, than in normal age-matched subjects [88]. Lindner and Scribner proposed the term « *accelerated atherosclerosis* » for this syndrome [89].

Among hemodialyzed patients, the incidence of atheromatous manifestations has increased in recent years, in parallel with the increasing age and longevity of patients treated by hemodialysis.

The principal causes of this « accelerated atherosclerosis » appear to be :

— the *level and duration of arterial hypertension* of the patient before starting hemodialysis, and above all, whether it persists after regular hemodialysis treatment. In our series, the incidence of severe vascular accidents was 3 percent in normotensive hemodialyzed subjects and 20 percent in those having persistent hypertension after the first six months of chronic hemodialysis [86];

— *lipid disorders* (particularly hypertriglyceridemia), secondary to uremia, often persisting during dialysis [90]. Attention has recently been drawn to the importance of this disorder [9];

— the *age* of the patient : spontaneous atherosclerosis, which has an increasing incidence in patients over 50 years of age, can be associated with the « accelerated atherosclerosis » due to uremia itself. Similarly, other factors, such as diabetes or tobacco, can contribute to this complication;

— the presence of *calcification of the arterial media,* induced by secondary hyperparathyroidism and increased phosphocalcic product, can aggravate arterial wall degeneration.

Coronary insufficiency is the most frequent clinical localization of diffuse vascular atherosclerosis observed in uremic patients. Its manifestations are often seen even before starting hemodialysis, particularly in aged patients. Angor can be increased during dialysis sessions and anemia plays a major role in inducing the complication. Angina usually appears in a patient when hematocrit falls below a critical level, and regular transfusions are often required for these patients. Myocardial infarction occurs three times more frequently in hemodialyzed patients over 50 years of age than in those under 30. It is still an unavoidable cause of death, as are cerebrovascular complications which will be discussed below [92].

Arteritis of the lower limbs is less frequent (except in diabetic patients) and in any case is not usually life-threatening.

8.1.3. Pericarditis

Pericarditis is a relatively frequent complication of chronic hemodialysis, seen in 20 to 25 percent of patients [93]. According to the time of occurrence relative to the initiation of dialysis treatment it may be termed « early » or « late ».

Early pericarditis occurs during the weeks immediately preceding or following the first dialysis. It is the most frequent type of pericarditis. It appears to be essentially induced by water and sodium overload [94]. Clinical manifestations are thoracic pain, pericardial friction rub and an increase in cardio-thoracic index. Treatment includes immediate beginning (or intensification) of hemodialysis, using careful local heparinization, and drastic water and sodium depletion, up to 10 percent of initial body weight.

Peritoneal dialysis can temporarily be used. This treatment almost always induces regression of the effusion (fig. 11). A hemopericardium with acute tamponade which requires

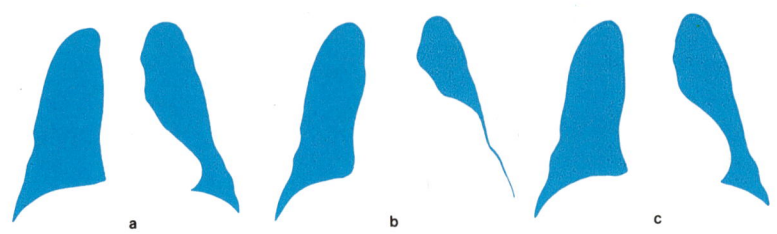

Fig. 11 - Uremic pericarditis, chest film :
a) Before inset of pericarditis. b) At the height of pericardial effusion. c) Following intensive dialysis and active fluid removal.

surgical drainage of the pericardium is relatively rare, observed in only 8 percent of our series. Recurrence is also rare, about 10 percent of cases [95].

Late pericarditis is defined as occurring after the first month of chronic dialysis treatment or later. Pathogenic factors are less clearly defined : water and sodium overload is frequent but not constant ; « inadequate » dialysis or vascular access thrombosis precedes pericarditis in many cases [95]. Pericardial friction rub and rapidly increasing cardiomegaly usually are sufficiently suggestive of diagnosis, but echocardiographic exmination is very useful for evaluating the volume of pericardial effusion and its evolution, and for excluding cardiomegaly of a different nature, particularly left ventricular dilatation and or hypertrophy.

Treatment includes intensification of dialysis with careful local heparinization, associated or not with antiinflammatory drugs such as corticosteroids or *indometacin* (Indocid®). Most often, this treatment reduces pericardial effusion within 10 to 15 days. However, in about one third of cases, the course can be a compressive hemopericardium. *Surgical drainage* of the pericardium then appears to be safer and more effective than pericardiocentesis [94].

8.1.4. Endocarditis

Acute endocarditis can appear after infection of vascular access, whether this be a shunt, internal fistula or a graft. Severe metastatic infections can occur, notably valvular lesions [96]. Cure requires prolonged antibiotic treatment and sacrifice of the infected vascular access.

8.1.5. Heart failure

Heart failure can be due to several mechanisms in the dialyzed patient :

— *left ventricular insufficiency* most often is secondary to poorly controlled arterial hypertension. It is often aggravated, sometimes bruskly, by excessive water and salt intake between dialyses. Its manifestations are acute pulmonary edema, which can be corrected by rapid ultrafiltration and immediate lowering of arterial pressure. Left ventricular insufficiency can also be ischemic in origin, secondary to coronary artery disease :

— *high-output cardiac failure* can be secondary to anemia (reflected by intense and extended mesocardiac murmur), or sometimes to an excessive flow rate in the fistula. In the later case, it may be improved by surgical reduction of the fistula blood flow rate ;

— *congestive uremic cardiomyopathy* presents usually as a severe cardiac failure, unexplained by any of the preceding factors. It is probably rare and its cause is still unknown; we have explored about 10 cases [97]. Congestive cardiomyopathy can be definitely diagnosed only when based on precise angiographic and hemodynamic criteria: it resembles primary congestive cardiomyopathy. Prognosis is severe, but reversal of the myocardial disorder following renal transplantation has been recently described [98].

8.2. Hematological problems

Uremia is responsible for erythrocyte, leukocyte and platelet alteration [99].

8.2.1. Anemia

Anemia is one of the major problems in hemodialyzed patients. It is enhanced by three factors:

— *insufficient medullary production,* secondary to deficient renal secretion or activation of erythropoietin [100]. It results that anemia is most severe in anephric patients, where hematocrit is often below 20 percent. On the other hand, in some kidney diseases such as polycystic disease, normal or only moderately decreased erythropoietin secretion may persist associated with moderate anemia or no anemia at all. Two other factors are also incriminated: 1) the possible inhibitory effect of uremic toxins on erythropoiesis and 2) invasion of the erythropoietic marrow by fibrous tissue during severe secondary hyperparathryroidism [101].

Despite deficient erythropoietin levels, red blood cell production can be improved by a good nutritional level, which increases the intake of essential aminoacids and vitamins. On the other hand, adequate dialysis increases the removal of toxins which would inhibit erythropoietin production:

— *increased endogenous hemolysis* by uremic toxins. Methylguanidine [102] and guanidinoproprionic acid have been particularly incriminated. In some cases, hemolysis results from hypersplenism, or occasionally from hypophosphatemia caused by an excessive use of phosphate binders. Hemolysis can also be caused by chloramines, nitrites or copper in the dialysate fluid [43];

— *blood loss* caused by hemodialysis treatment itself, such as blood sampling for laboratory investigations, incomplete return of blood after dialysis sessions, or coagulations within the dialyzer. These blood losses can be increased by gastrointestinal bleeding, or menorrhagia, which are enhanced by poor hemostasis.

Anemia is the main cause of the weakness felt by dialysis patients. It can be the only cause of a lack of rehabilitation. In patients suffering from coronary insufficiency, it increases the incidence of stenocardiac pain.

Treatment

Simultaneous action must be taken whenever it is possible:

— *blood samplings* should be reduced; blood should be carefully returned at the end of dialysis sessions;

— *iron supplements* should be administered whenever blood level drops below 100 mcg/100 ml, preferably orally, but intravenous administration is also possible;

— *splenectomy* may rarely be indicated in incontrollable anemia requiring repeated transfusions, when isotopic examination proves reduced red blood cell half-life and splenic hypersequestration;

— administration of *androgens* is debated: long-term usefulness has not been established [104], administration in the female induces virilization, and in both sexes it increases plasma lipid disorders.

Transfusions may be necessary when anemia is poorly tolerated, as manifested by dyspnea, extreme asthenia, subintrant angor, or in case of acute bleeding. However, transfusions further inhibit residual erythropoietin secretion. In addition, an elevated number of transfusions entails hemosiderosis, which is difficult to halt. It is thus recommended not to transfuse young patients who have no ischemic complications and whose asthenia is not too severe.

However, the present medical *attitude toward transfusing* patients who may eventually be transplanted is no longer as restrictive as it used to be. Whereas in some patients transfusions produce cytotoxic antibodies directed against HLA specificities, (enhancing subsequent graft rejection), in others transfusion appears to produce « facilitating » antibodies. This is probably the explanation for the recent observation that functional graft survival rate is higher in patients having been transfused but not having antibodies directed against HLA specificites, than in those never having been transfused. In present practice, any dialysis patient who requires transfusion can be transfused; the possible subsequent appearance of anti-HLA antibodies should be checked after each transfusion. Patients who do not develop such antibodies, despite repeated transfusions, are particularly good subjects for transplantation. On the other hand, patients who do develop these antibodies can be transplanted only from a donor who does not have the corresponding antigens.

8.2.2. Leukocyte alterations

The number of leukocytes is normal or slightly reduced in the uremic patient; a certain degree of lymphopenia which seems to accompany the reduction in T cells related to the immune defect seen in uremic patients, is observed. During dialysis, a large decrease in the number of circulating leukocytes is seen; it attains a maximum drop at about the 15th minute and returns to normal at about the first hour. This phenomenon seems due to *leukocyte sequestration* on the dialysis membrane [105] as well as to pulmonary sequestration, resulting from complement activation by cellophane membranes [106].

In case of infection, leukocytosis with polynucleosis develops at normal levels in the uremic patient.

8.2.3. Platelet alterations

In the hemodialyzed patient, the number of platelets is usually normal. However platelet functions are altered in end-stage renal insufficiency, with longer bleeding time, decrease in platelet adherence to glass and aggregation of platelets induced by ADP or collagen, and reduction in factor 3 platelets activity [107]. These disorders are responsible for at least part of the hemorrhagic tendency observed in these patients.

Platelet functional alterations probably are related to dialyzable toxins such as guanidinosuccinic acid [108] or phenols [109]. They are quickly corrected by the first dialysis sessions. Thus, assessing platelet functions has been proposed for evaluating hemodialysis adequacy.

8.3. Neurologic complications

The neurological complications seen in dialysis patients stem from two principal mechanisms: retention of neurotoxic metabolites, and secondary atheromatous vascular

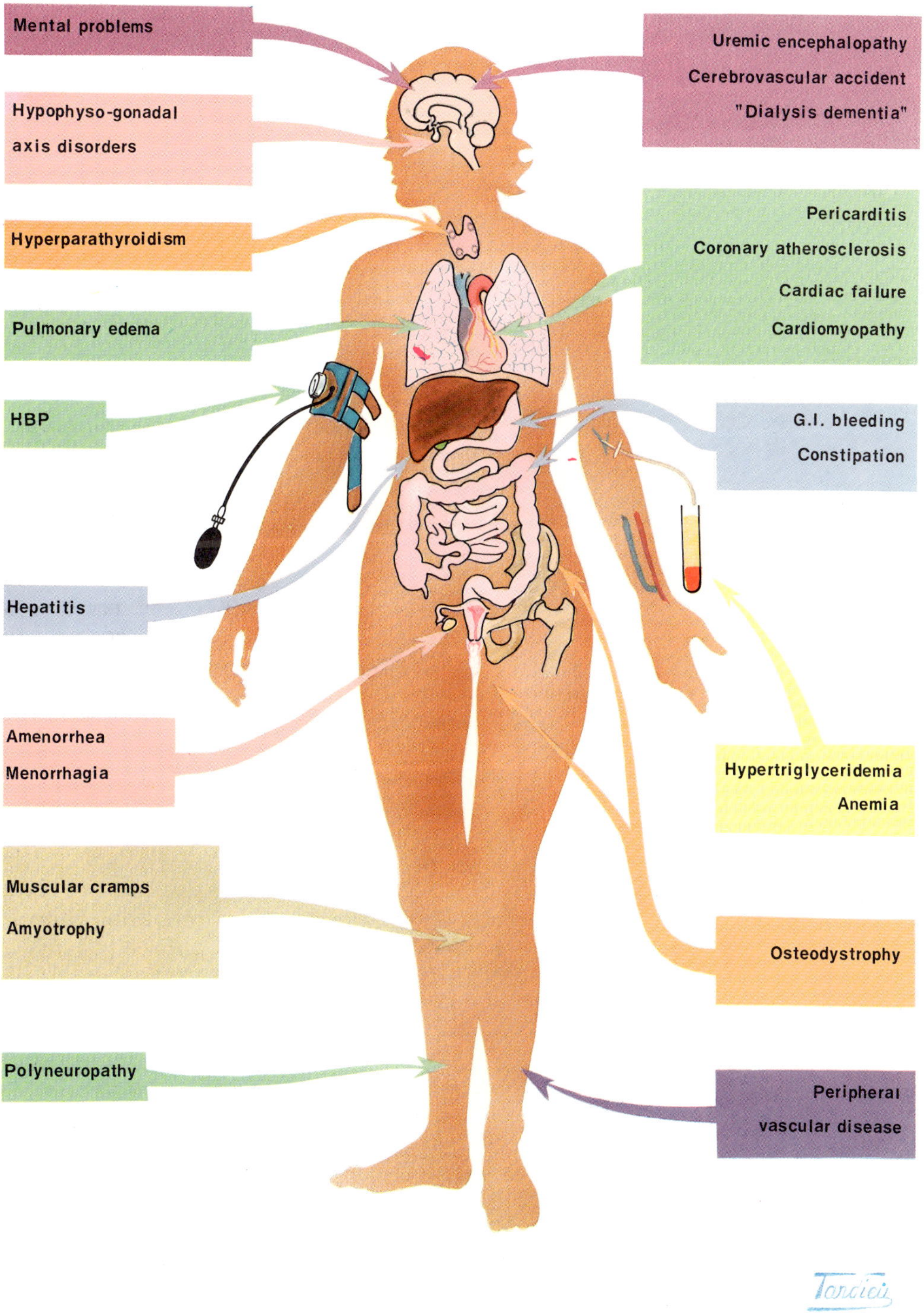

VISCERAL AND METABOLIC DISORDERS OF CHRONIC UREMIA

Pl. 22

- Mental problems
- Hypophyso-gonadal axis disorders
- Hyperparathyroidism
- Pulmonary edema
- HBP
- Hepatitis
- Amenorrhea / Menorrhagia
- Muscular cramps / Amyotrophy
- Polyneuropathy

- Uremic encephalopathy / Cerebrovascular accident / "Dialysis dementia"
- Pericarditis / Coronary atherosclerosis / Cardiac failure / Cardiomyopathy
- G.I. bleeding / Constipation
- Hypertriglyceridemia / Anemia
- Osteodystrophy
- Peripheral vascular disease

involvement. In addition, some complications appear directly linked to hemodialysis treatment itself [110].

8.3.1. Disorders related to uremic toxicity

a. *Uremic encephalopathy* : this term describes functional alterations of the central nervous system secondary to the accumulation of uremic toxins. Manifestations are behavioral disorders : physical and intellectual asthenia, difficulty in concentration, irritability, anxiety, nocturnal insomnia and somnolence during the day. Later appear disorientation, memory disorders, confusion and progressive torpor. Neuro-muscular disorders are also seen : cramps, trembling and generalized muscular twitching. The EEG shows disorganization of the basic alpha rhythm, with succeeding groups of slow waves. These disorders rapidly and completely regress with dialysis. This would suggest a responsibility of low molecular weight toxins, probably organic acids [110].

Semi-quantitative methods of measuring intellectual performance and EEG tracing have been suggested to evaluate dialysis efficacy [111].

b. *Uremic polyneuritis* : this term describes a symmetrical sensori-motor polyneuritis, predominantly of the extremities of the inferior limbs, but which can be extended to the upper limbs as well. First are seen sensory alterations such as paresthesias, often as « burning feet » or prickling sensations, painful cramps and muscular « impatience » usually occurring during the night and which can be only be calmed by movement (« restless legs syndrome »). Later appears a decrease in osteotendon reflexes and, in severe forms, motor disorders with tiredness when walking, and steppage gait which may reach flaccid paraplegia [112]. The *autonomous system* is often also affected, as seen by orthostatic hypotension and difficulty in obtaining erection [113].

Diagnosis is confirmed by decrease in *motor nerve-conduction velocity* (MNCV), which normally is higher than 40 m/second at the common popliteal nerve. However, variations in MNCV appear and disappear slowly. Thus, this examination cannot detect short term polyneuritis but can only be used to assess long-term dialysis efficacity [114]. The vibratory perception threshhold has been suggested as a simpler and quicker technique for detecting polyneuritis [115].

Aside from its clinical consequences this complication has theroretical interest, for it is at the basis of Babb and Scribner's hypothesis concerning middle molecules. These authors suggested that polyneuritis could be due to insufficient removal of neurotoxic solutes having a molecular weight over 1,000 daltons. It has been seen that polyneuritis does not occur when the rules for adequate dialysis based upon sufficient removal of middle molecules are carefully respected, and that polyneuritis can be reversed when dialysis is intensified, particularly by te use of high permeability membranes. Clinical improvement is seen, although marked decrease in nerve transmission velocity can long remain.

Possible vitamin deficiency due to dialysis losses has never been proven and does not seem probable ; massive administration of vitamin B does not change the course of polyneuritis.

8.3.2. Neurologic complications related to chronic hemodialysis

a. *Cerebrovascular accidents*

Hemorrhagic cerebrovascular accidents (meningeal or cerebromeningeal hemorrhage) are often lethal. They occur more frequently in hemodialyzed patients than in uremic patients not yet dialyzed, suggesting a role of anticoagulants. Their etiology is the same as that of coronary insufficiency. Arterial hypertension plays a principal role. In our series, these accidents occurred almost exclusively in patients who remained hypertensive after the 6th month of dialysis [86]. They are seen more frequently in patients over 50 years of age [92].

b. *Subdural hematoma*

Subdural hematoma is not exceptional in dialysis patients. The bleeding, which occurs between the dura and the arachnoid, is probably induced by too rapid extracellular dehydration aggravated by heparinization. During hemodialysis, it is manifested by headache, dizziness, vomiting and then coma with signs of localization. The signs persist despite interruption of dialysis, and progressively worsen [116]. Diagnosis is difficult, but essential, because only early surgical drainage can save the patient. Subdural hematoma should be distinguished from cerebral infarction which only requires suspension of heparinization for 3 to 4 weeks, temporary peritoneal dialysis often being used.

c. *Dialysis disequilibrium syndrome*

Rapid hemodialysis can bring on headache, nausea, vomiting, hypertension, cramps, shaking, agitation, trembling, disorientation, generalized convulsions and then coma. These disorders are usually reversible within several hours following the end of dialysis. The *cerebrospinal fluid* is always hypertensive [117]. These disorders usually occur when blood urea concentration exceeds 300 mg/100 ml. This suggests a gradient between the osmotic concentration in the brain and in the plasma because of the slow diffusion of urea out of the cellular compartment. However, it is not certain that only urea is responsible for osmotic hypertonia in the brain. Recent works suggest a role of intracerebral accumulation of organic acids which have not yet been identified [117]. Other authors have suggested that an increase in hemoglobin affinity for oxygen during dialysis, enhanced by correction of acidosis, could provoke tissular, and particularly cerebral, hypoxia.

Emergency treatment of these accidents includes intravenous infusion of solutes to temporarily increase plasma osmolarity, such as glucose, or better, mannitol or glycerol. In practice, such accidents should rather be avoided by progressively initiating dialysis in the first few sessions [117].

d. *Dialysis encephalopathy, or « dialysis dementia »*

A strange encephalopathy was described in 1972 in a dialysis center in Denver [118]. First appeared dysarthria, dysmetria, trembling, myoclonias, memory and characterical disorders, hallucinations, and then dementia and convulsions, leading to death in about 6 months, despite intensification of dialyss treatment. The only anomaly discovered in all of these patients was an abnormally high aluminum content of the cerebral gray matter.

Similar observations have been made in other centers. In each case, elevated plasma levels of aluminum have also been observed.

An etiological role of prolonged high doses of aluminum hydroxyde is suggested in several observations [118]. In other cases, excessive aluminum content of city water, and thus of the dialysate, has been proven [119]. Possibly, in some cases, these two factors are associated.

8.3.3. Neurological accidents of iatrogenic origin

Drugs which are usually eliminated by the kidney accumulate in the plasma and tissues of the uremic patient and to an even greater extent in the patient already on hemodialysis. In the dialysis patient these drugs are removed only to a small degree by hemodialysis. While the nephrotoxicity of the drugs is unimportant in these patients, neurological and sensorial effects can occur [120].

Some *antibacterial agents*, such as aminosides, can affect the eight cranial pair with deafness (Streptomycine, Kanamycine, Vancomycine) or vestibular disorders (Gentamicin, Tobramycin). Colimycin can cause neuropsychic disorders. Ethambutol and Isoniazide can provoke encephalic disorders or polyneuritis. When these antibiotics must be given to a patient on dialysis, strict rules of dosage adjustement must be followed.

When *sedatives* are overdosed, neuropsychic accidents can occur, with diffuse extrapyramidal contractures, particularly involving muscles of the face, the mouth and the tongue. Muscular twitching can follow, leading to hypotonic coma, with occasional convulsions and respiratory depression. The most frequently incriminated drugs are the benzodiazepines, the phenothiazines and barbiturics with a long half-life. A similar effect is seen for metoclopramide (Primperan®) which is often prescribed for nausea or vomiting.

8.3.4. Mental problems

Minor mental problems occur frequently in the advanced uremic state. They are partly due to uremic toxicity. An anxiety reaction is often seen in the dialysis patient with regard to possible technical accidents. A *depressive tendency* can be associated; it can be expressed as aggressivity toward the patient's surroundings or disinterest in diet and treatment. It is usually a reaction to the inevitable constraint of dialysis and the social and professional problems dialysis can incur (loss of job or inability to lead a normal life). Regular conversations with the patient are necessary to allow him to express these frustrations and to help him overcome them.

Major psychiatric problems are rare (melancolic depression, hypomania, refusal to continue dialysis, or even suicide attempts). They can require the assistance of a psychiatrist. Chimiotherapy is often beneficial.

8.4. Disorders of phospho-calcic metabolism

Phosphate and calcium metabolism disorders complicating hemodialysis may be recognized only during regular dialysis treatment. Most often, in fact, they occur in chronic uremia when appropriate treatment has not been provided [121].

Mechanisms (plate 23)

A primary disorder is a *defect in 25 (OH) vitamin D_3 conversion* to 1, 25 $(OH)_2$ vitamin D_3 by diseased kidneys [122]. An insufficiency of this active metabolite reduces intestinal absorption of calcium and leads to hypocalcemia. Hypocalcemia stimulates parathyroid glands secretion. On the other hand, the *hyperphosphatemia* which results from the renal tubular excretion defect also stimulates parathyroid secretion by decreasing plasma concentration of ionized calcium [123]. This secondary hyperparathyroidism is all the more elevated as it encounters target cell resistance, particularly that of osteoclasts, to parathyroid hormone action. Lastly, it is increased by reduction of kidney degradation of active hormone fragments [124]. The role of thyrocalcitonin is not clearly elucidated; its plasma concentration is usually increased.

The end result of all these disorders is bone demineralization, evidenced by quantitative bone biopsies. Hyperparathyroid lesions (*fibrous osteitis*) predominate; they are generally characterized by hyperosteolysis and medullary fibrosis, which reduces the volume of the erythropoietic marrow. *Osteomalacic lesions* are often associated, marked by excess osteoid tissue and shrinkage of calcification fronts. Considerable geographic

CALCIUM AND PHOSPHATE DISORDERS

Pl. 23

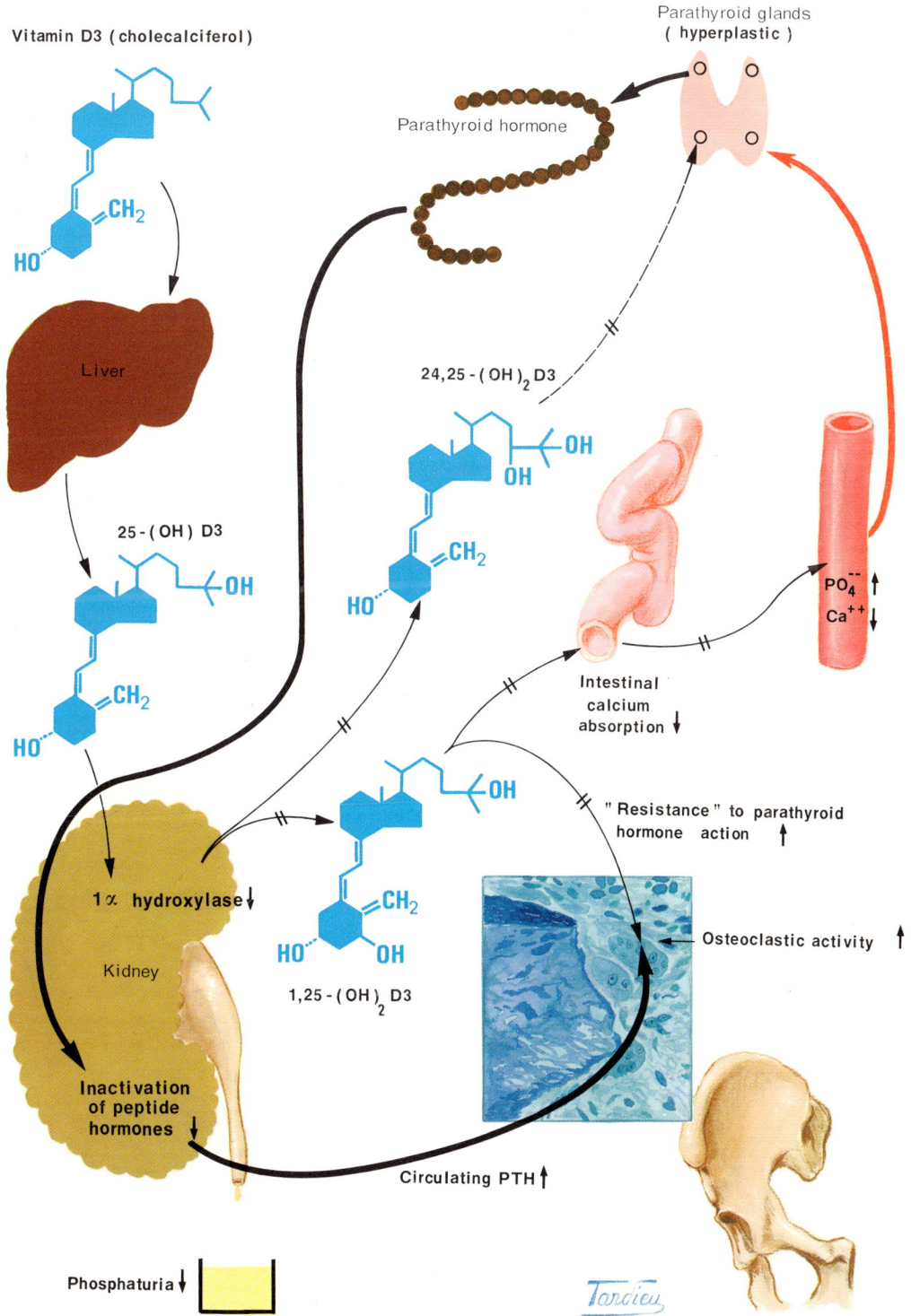

variations in the incidence and predominant type of bone disease exist ; differences in body stores of 25 hydroxcholecalciferol, secondary to various exposures to sunlight, may play a part [124].

It appears that hyperparathyroid resorption reacts electively to 1 alpha, 25 (OH)$_2$ vitamin D$_3$ and osteomalacic lesions to 25 OH vitamin D$_3$ [122].

Clinical and laboratory manifestations

In dialysis patients, calcemia is usually between 8.5 and 10.0 mg/100 ml due to calcium transfer during dialysis. Phosphate level is usually between 3.0 and 5.0 mg/100 ml, due to the associated effect of dialysis and inhibitors of intestinal phosphorus absorption. In some cases, hypercalcemia occurs. More often, insufficient control of phosphatemia is seen, reaching or exceeding 10.0 mg/100 ml. In these cases, the phosphocalcic product can exceed 75.

Certain clinical manifestations reflect *phosphocalcic product elevation,* such as a untractable *pruritus,* leading to lesions induced by scratching which are a source of infection ; pararticulary *metatastatic calcifications,* responsible for « pseudo-gout » ; calcification of soft tissues, or of arterial walls, visualized on pelvic X-rays or X-rays of the hands.

Bone complications can lead to rachidian pain or even diffuse bone pain or spontaneous fractures. *Radiographic signs* of hyperparathyroidism are subperiostal resorption of the phalanges and resorption of the external extremities of the clavicles. Lesions suggesting osteomalacia also are seen, such as fissures in the ischio-pubian branches or the ribs. Rarely, osteoporosis is associated. Only bone biopsy can assess the respective importance of fibrous osteitis and osteomalacia and evaluate the effect of treatment.

Treatment

The treatment of phosphocalcic disorders today is mostly prophylactic.

In the chronic uremic patient, blood calcium should be maintained between 9.0 and 10.0 mg/100 ml with calcium supplement, or if necessary with 25 (OH) vitamin D$_3$ (Dedrogyl®). Blood phosphorus should be maintained between 4.0 and 5.0 mg/100 ml with intestinal phosphate binders.

In the hemodialyzed patient, the same is true. Blood calcium level should be maintained between 8.5 and 10.0 mg/100 ml by calcium supplements if necessary.

Maintaining plasma phosphate within optimal limits, i.e. 4.0 to 5.0 mg/100 ml, is essential.

It is achieved by phosphate binders such as aluminum hydroxyde or other preparations, taken about 1 hour after meals. However, excessive correction of phosphatemia should be avoided, since it can induce hypophosphatemia causing encephalic disorders, or osteomalacia.

The synthesis of *vitamin D derivatives* has provided considerable improvement in the treatment of these disorders. They are now used to decrease parathyroid hypersecretion and to normalize bone metabolism : 1 alpha, 25 (OH)$_2$D$_3$ (or its synthetic analogue, 1 alpha, (OH) D$_3$) reduces fibrous osteitis [125] [126] ; 25 (OH) D$_3$ is believed to electively stimulate mineralization of osteoid tissue ; it is preferred for combatting the osteomalacic component [127]. However, lesions of renal osteodystrophy are often mixed, and an association of the two derivatives is probably often useful.

In some cases, parathyroid hypersecretion is so high that it induces severe bone lesions which cannot be halted by vitamin supplements without dangerous hypercalcemia and/or hyperphosphatemia. Subtotal or total *parathyroidectomy* may then be necessary. It can be followed or not by reimplantation of parathyroid fragments in the forearm. Nevertheless, early medical treatment should make surgery less necessary in the future.

8.5. Infectious problems

In hemodialyzed patients, infection is enhanced by an immune defect, which is common to uremic patients and incompletely corrected by chronic hemodialysis. This defect particularly involves cell mediated immunity and it explains the frequent negative skin reactions to tuberculin. The frequent vitamin B_6 (pyridoxin) deficiency of dialyzed patients no doubt contributes to functional alteration of T lymphocytes [128].

Bacterial or viral contamination results from technically imperfect dialysis, poor technique in creating vascular access, manipulations for dialysis, or contamination among dialysis patients in centers.

8.5.1. Bacterial infections

Bacterial infections involve mainly the vascular access, particularly shunts. The most frequent cause is the staphylococcus, a skin germ which is common in hemodialysis patients, particularly in cases of prurit. Other infectious localizations are usually secondary, by diffusion through the blood stream. These can be pulmonary, bone or meningeal localizations, or acute bacterial endocarditis. Their cure requires suppression of the primary infectious site.

Urinary infection poses a special problem in the case of hemodialyzed patients with polycystic kidneys, lithiasis or infectious uropathy. It is enhanced by oliguria and can be reflected by acute pyelonephritis or even pyonephrosis, requiring *nephrectomy*. The urinary infection can be responsible for a gram-negative septicemia.

8.5.2. Tuberculosis infections

Tuberculosis occurs in dialyzed patients approximately 10 times more frequently than in the general population. It may be pulmonary, lymphatic, bone or meningeaal. It often presents with a long, unexplained fever. Skin reactions to tuberculin are only inconstantly positive, even in the most active forms.

8.5.3 Virus B hepatitis (pl. 24)

Center patients are often carriers of the antigen associated with hepatitis B virus (HBsAg); home patients are less affected [129].

Doctors, nurses and technicians in hospitals often contract virus B hepatitis. In dialysis patients, hepatitis is usually anicteric and is detectable by moderate elevation of transaminases and appearance of HBs Ag [130]. The antigen has a tendency to persist indefinitely in many of these patients, which helps spread the infection [131]. The course is almost always benign, and the development of cirrhosis is infrequent.

Contamination of the staff is a serious problem, and several cases of severe hepatitis have occurred during recent years [6]. It points up the necessity for strict hygiene in dialysis centers. It should be noted that such strict measures have resulted in removing practically all hepatitis from centers in Great Britain [132].

Passive immunization with specific gamma-globulins has reduced the incidence of hepatitis among staff and patients [133]. Active immunization is under study.

8.5.4. Prolonged fever

In some cases, bacterial or viral infectious complications in dialysis patients present as unexplained fever of long-duration. Principal causes of long-duration fever in dialysis patients are shown below.

Infection of vascular access
Thrombosis of the fistula or of the arteriovenous shunt
Pericarditis
Nose, throat, ear or buccal infection
Pleuro-pulmonary infection, either viral or bacterial
Urinary infection
Viral hepatitis
Pulmonary or extrapulmonary tuberculosis
Febrile surgical emergencies
Exceptionnaly, periarteritis associated with hepatitis B virus

---

8.6. Metabolic and endocrine problems

8.6.1. Metabolic disorders

a) *Carbohydrate metabolism*

In end-stage uremia, an intolerance for glucose appears. It is characterized by a paradiabetic glycemic curve following oral glucose lod. It is not corrected by chronic hemodialysis. An increase is also seen in criculating insulin and glucagon levels, secondary both to excessive secretion and reduced renal degradation. They occur because of perturbations of glycolysis and neoglucogenesis as well as resistance to the action of insuline and hypersensitivity to that of glucagon [134].

b) *Lipid metabolism*

The importance of disorders of lipid metabolism in uremic patients has recently been pointed out [88]. It involves hypertriglyceridemia associated with an elevation of prebetalipoproteins, which would play a role at the origin of the « accelerated atherosclerosis » observed in the uremic patient [90]. The *reduction of carbohydrates* and substitution of *unsaturated fats* for saturated fats can often partially diminish hypertriglyceridemia [135]. In cases of severe hypertriglyceridemia, clofibrate treatment may be useful; dosage should be reduced in function of its reduced excretion.

c) *Vitamin and nutritional disorders*

Vitamin deficiency is observed in dialysis patients. It results in part from loss of hydrosoluble vitamins during dialysis. Nevertheless, the deficit is usually compensated by intake,

HEPATITIS B: INFECTION IN HEMODIALYSIS CENTERS

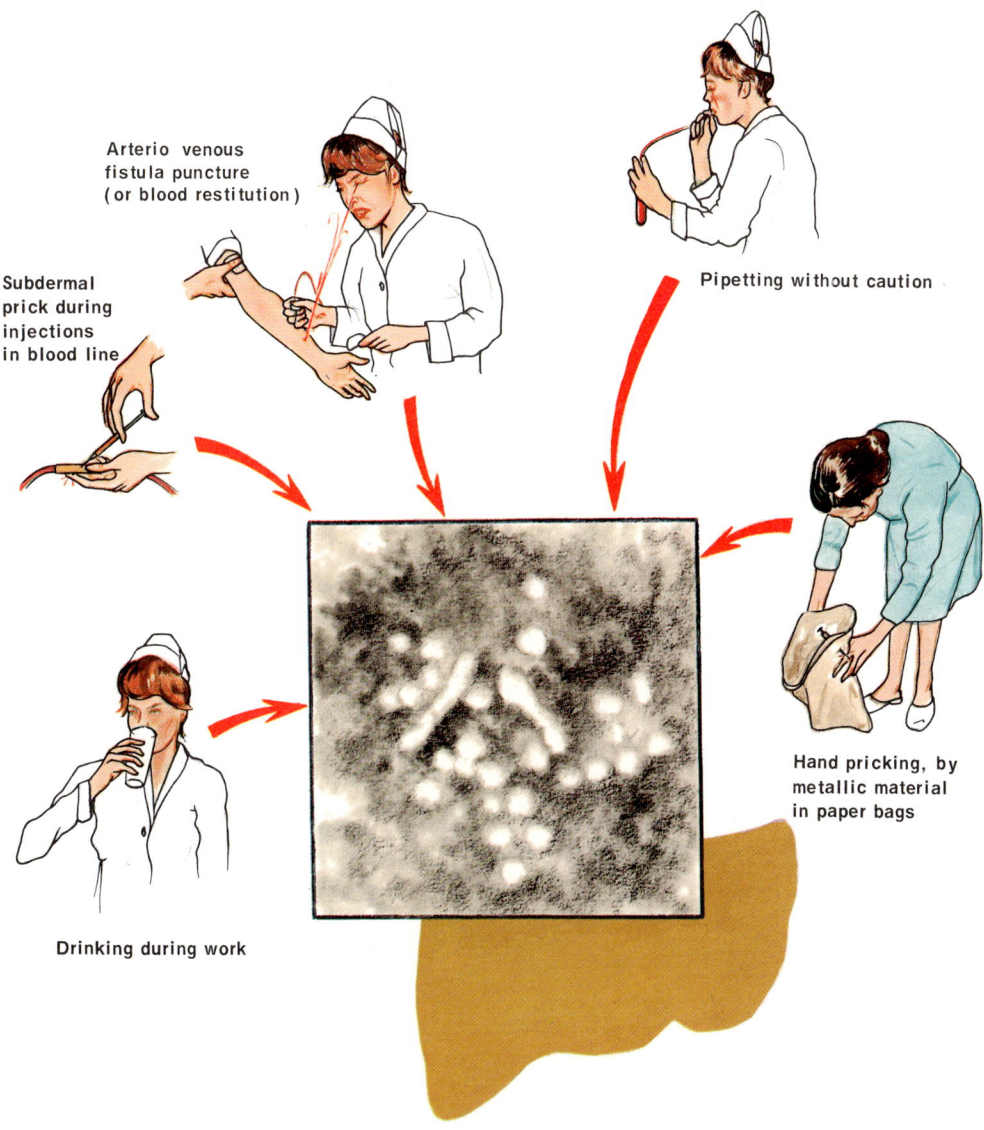

Arterio venous fistula puncture (or blood restitution)

Subdermal prick during injections in blood line

Pipetting without caution

Drinking during work

Hand pricking, by metallic material in paper bags

Electron microscopy of B virus in plasma, showing circular (isolated or clustered) and also tubular forms and no clinical manifestations have been proven to be due to vitamin deficiency. However, in patients suffering from anorexia a possible deficiency should be prevented by supplementation with 1 mg folic acid, 100 mg ascorbic acid and 300 mg pyridoxine.

A certain degree of *malnutrition,* characterized by reduction of the muscular mass, is often observed in dialysis patients. It cannot be explained by the loss of aminoacids during dialysis because this loss does not exceed 5 to 10 gram per session and is easily replaced by food intake. It is probably rather due to alterations of intermediate nitrogen metabolism and to reduced synthesis of muscular proteins, secondary to glucagon hypersecretion and to peripheric resistance to insulin [136].

8.6.2. Endocrine disorders

Numerous endocrine problems, associated with uremia, have been described.

1) The levels of circulating *thyroid hormones* are moderately decreased, without signs of hypothyroidism.

2) Alterations of the *hypophyso-gonadal axis,* on the contrary, present a clinical problem.

— *In the male,* plasma testosterone is often decreased in parallel to the increase in circulating gonadostimulin levels; an insufficient response to stimulation by chorionic gonadotrophins is frequent. Oligospermia with hypomotility of the spermatozoids is frequent, but fertility may not be affected. Libido and sexual activity are often reduced in the dialysis patient, but this also depends on the degree of asthenia due to anemia [137].

— *In the fermale, amenorrhea* is often seen in advanced uremia. It is associated with non elevated FSH and LH levels. Stimulation by LH-RH brings normal hypophyseal response, demonstrating the suprahypophyseal origin of the disorder [138]. During the first months following dialysis, menstrual periods usually reappear. Then they often are complicated by menorrhagia. FSH and LH are seen to be normal; progesterone is sometimes normally elevated during the luteal period, reflecting ovulation, but it mostly remains low. This *luteal defect* explains in part the menorrhagia. Rather than total suppression of menstrual periods, substitute luteinizing treatment is indicated for normalizing menstrual cycles and avoiding blood loss during dialysis.

8.7. Gastrointestinal problems

Anorexia, nausea and vomiting are frequent when blood urea exceeds 300 mg/100 ml. They are augmented by hyponatremia. These disorders disappear with chronic hemodialysis but can recur during infectious complications or antibiotic treatment.

Constipation is frequent in patients taking aluminum gels to inhibit intestinal absorption of phosphate. It can be improved by Sorbitol®, Mucilages or paraffine.

Gastralgias, resulting from gastritis or duodenitis are sometimes seen. Hiatal hernias appear more frequently in dialysis patients than in the general population, but gastroduodenal ulcer is rare, despite the frequent increase in gastric acid secretion and gastrinemia. Aluminum derivatives, which are used for the control of blood phosphate, are also indicated in this case for their antacid effect.

Uncontrollable *ascitis,* exudative, is sometimes seen. It can occur after peritoneal dialysis; more often, is it due to water and sodium overload or portal hypertension. It is questionable whether a « uremic » ascitis per se actually exists.

8.8. Surgery in the dialysis patient

> **Any form of surgery can be performed in the dialysis patient with proper precautions concerning anesthestics and hemostatis.**

Indications for surgery may be related to dialysis or primary nephropathy itself: nephrectomy for severe urinary infection or repeated hematuria, particularly in polycystic disease; preparation for a transplant; binephrectomy for uncontrollable hypertension. It can also be indicated by complications stemming from dialysis, such as pericardial drainage, subtotal parathyroidectomy, splenectomy, creation of vascular access, or by surgical emergency outside of dialysis, such as appendectomy or cholecystectomy.

Certain *precautions* must be taken with the dialysis patient who is to undergo surgery.

— The surgery should never take place less than 6 to 8 hours after dialysis, for elimination of all residual heparin. This last presurgical hemodialysis will reduce functional platelet disorders resulting from uremia and correct electrolyte imbalance, particularly hyperkalemia and acidosis. Additional ultrafiltration should be performed [50] as to leave the anesthetist the possibility of using perfusions or transfusions if necessary during surgery.

— Anesthesia should be performed by a well-trained team. Analgesics can be used at normal doses, but the choice of neuromuscular blocking agents is very important. Some derivatives having a short half-life (bromure of pancuronium or d-tubocurarine) should be used, and at reduced doses. Vascular access must be carefully protected and checked during and after surgical procedure.

— After surgery dialysis should not be performed before 36 to 48 hours. This will avoid bleeding in the area of surgery. The first dialyses should be performed with local heparinization.

8.9. Dialysis in high-risk patients

Special problems are present in aged patients or in those with systemic diseases.

8.9.1. Dialysis in elderly patients

Hemodialysis can be indicated in the elderly when the general and vascular state of the patient suggests the probability of prolonged survival with good possibilities or rehabilitation [139]. The tolerance of the treatment is usually good and home dialysis is often possible [4]. The principal problem stems from coronary insufficiency, requiring repeated transfusions, particularly during the first dialysis sessions. Serum potassium should be carefully controlled and generally requires dialysis baths with higher potassium content than usual.

8.9.2. Dialysis in patients with systemic disease

Chronic hemodialysis has now expanded to the point where a growing number of patients with kidney failure due to systemic disease are admitted to dialysis programs [6]. In these cases results depend on the visceral localizations and extension of the primary disease.

In *diabetic* patients, insulin requirement usually increases during dialysis treatment, and glycemic equilibrium is frequently difficult to attain [40]. Survival depends on the course of diabetic vascular lesions.

In patients with generalized *amylosis* or *multiple myeloma,* survival depends on the stage of the disease. On the contrary, survival is usually good in patients with systemic lupus erythematosus [4].

8.10. Dialysis in the child

Chronic hemodialysis can be used in the child. It is more difficult than in adults, from both technical and psychological points of view. Dialysis has been performed in children as young as two or three years [141].

8.10.1. Indications

Kidney diseases leading to terminal renal failure and requiring chronic hemodialysis are different in the child from those in the adult. Congenital nephropathies and malformative uropathies are the more frequent causes [142].

Criteria indicating the need for dialysis are the same, i.e., decrease of creatinine clearance below 5 ml/min/1.73 m^2. Plasma creatinine at this stage is lower than in the adult, thus the need for dialysis corresponds to 5.0 to 6.0 mg/100 ml in the young child [141].

8.10.2. Technical problems

— Creation of *vascular access* requires general anesthesia. Internal fistulae or arteriovenous grafts are more often used than arteriovenous shunts which last for a shorter time.

— *Dialysers* should contain an amount of extracorporeal blood which is in proportion to the child's weight, about 10 to 15 ml/kg. The rate of solute transfer should be reduced in order to avoid osmotic disequilibrium. Dialyzer urea clearance should not exceed 2 or 3 ml/mn/1.73 m^2. Parallel-plate dialyzers are the most used, with a limited number of circuits providing a reduced membrane surface area adapted to the child. Dialysers specially designed for pediatric use are also available.

— *Ultrafiltration rate* must be very carefully controlled. Continuous weight surveillance may be necessary in the young child. The same is true of clinical tolerance and blood pressure. A parent or friend must be continuously present during the whole session.

8.10.3. Results

Despite these difficulties, good *results* are generally attained. In 70 percent of cases, the child can again attend school normally. The daily diet should include 2 to 3 g/kg protein, of which two-thirds should be animal proteins, calcium supplements and active derivatives of vitamin D. Growth is usually retarded with a slowing of skeletal development. Hematocrit is often below 20 percent.

Principal *complications* during or between dialysis sessions are frequent convulsions and cardiac accidents. Nevertheless, overall survival is surprisingly good, reaching 90 percent at 5 years of dialysis treatment, in the series of the pediatric dialysis department of the Enfants-Malades Hospital in Paris [141].

IX. LIVING WITH HEMODIALYSIS

> The aim of chronic hemodialysis is to provide each patient the possibility of leading a life as close to normal as possible. Despite the constraints inherent in the treatment and the problems which have not yet been solved, this aim is reached in most cases, particularly those undergoing dialysis treatment at home.

9.1. Overall results of chronic hemodialysis

A high possibility of survival is offered by chronic hemodialysis treatment today. No theoretical limit exists for the survival of these patients. Several hundred dialysis patients have survived more than 10 years and some for more than 15 years.

The *overall survival* of these patients, expressed by the actuarial method, shows an annual mortality rate of less than 10 percent for all European centers [6]. Results are better in centers with longer experience. Regular dialysis treatment began at Necker Hospital in 1962. If the first two years are not considered (techniques were still quite rudimentary), the overall cumulative survival rate between 1964 and 1975 in Necker Hospital and associated centers is 84.3 percent at three years and 75.7 percent at five years, that is, a *mean annual mortality rate* of less than 5 percent [4]. The best results are seen in home dialysis patients, with actuarial survival of 79.5 percent at five years (fig. 12). Comparable résults have been seen in other centers with a similar expérience [6,65].

Moreover, the consequences of complications which can occur in dialysis patients must not be overestimated. In our recent experience a mean of only 10 *days of hospitalization* per patient per year was required [4].

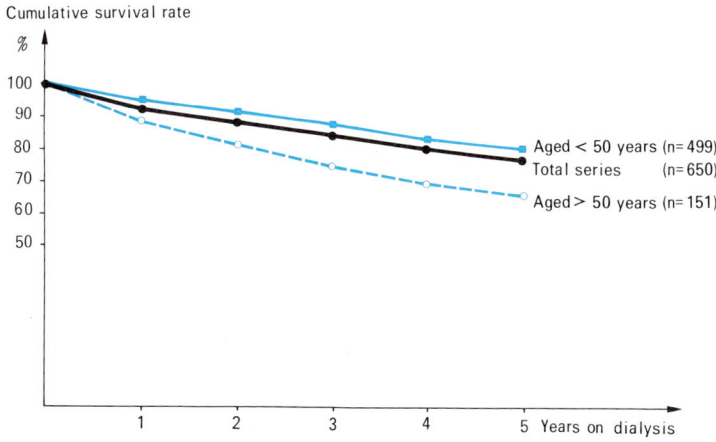

Fig. 12 - Cumulative survival of regular dialysis patients (Necker hospital and associated centers).

9.2. Diet of the hemodialyzed patient

> Chronic hemodialysis permits an increased daily intake of proteins, which usually meets with patient approval. On the other hand, restrictions in water and electrolyte intake must be accepted. Complementary treatments to control phosphocalcic metabolism are essential.

— *Protein intake* should be at least equal to 1 gm/kg/day in patients treated two times a week, but in those treated three times it can be unrestricted.

— *Liquid intake* ideally should not exceed 700 ml/day over residual diuresis. It should be regulated so that no more than 2 kg of body weight are gained by the patient between two dialyses.

— *Sodium chloride intake* is usually about 2 gm per day. It can be higher when residual diuresis is relatively elevated or in some binephrectomized patients with permanent arterial hypotension.

— Intake of foods rich in *potassium* must be restricted (fruits, vegetables, chocolate). To avoid overrestriction, which would be poorly tolerated, an ion exchange resin on each nondialysis day is useful in most patients.

— Blood *calcium* level requires calcium carbonate intake of 2 to 4 gm daily. Supplementation with synthetic derivatives of vitamin D is often necessary.

— Plasma *phosphate* level control is very important. The high protein diet brings a permanent tendency to hyperphosphatemia and requires sufficient intake of aluminum hydroxyde (4 to 8 gm/day) or similar preparations. Overdoses should be avoided. The level of plasma aluminum should be regularly checked.

9.3. The quality of life of the dialyzed patient

The dietetic and therapeutic requirements for the patient on dialysis are limiting, but when they complement adequate dialysis, life can be quite close to normal.

The main problem for center-treated patients is the rigidity of their dialysis schedule. Home patients can choose the days and hours which best suit them and their family.

For adolescents, dependence on dialysis and diet seems to be particularly ill-tolerated. In that case, transplantation is the method of choice. Tolerance is best in adult patients with good, supportive family environment.

Dialysis patients should be able to take *vacations*. Several solutions exist, such as holiday centers for dialyzed children, self-dialysis centers for travelling home dialysis patients or simply exchange between centers. Precautions should be taken to avoid the spread of virus B hepatitis by carriers to centers which are not contaminated.

9.4. Social and professional rehabilitation

> Resuming (or maintaining) normal professional activity is not only economically necessary for most dialysis patients, but it is also psychologically important. Full-time professional activity is more often possible when dialysis is performed at home. It can also be possible for in-center patients when employers accept to arrange their working hours. This is often the case when they are properly informed.

In our experience, about 60 percent of in-center patients resume full- or part-time activity; this figure reaches 80 percent for those treated at home [4][6]. The fact that more than 20 percent of currently treated patients have reached retirement age should be taken into account in judging these results.

Professional rehabilitation is sometimes difficult because of business and government reticence to employing the « handicapped ». Better informing of the public has reduced this problem to a certain degree. Today most well-informed employers assist by adapting hours and working conditions of these employees.

9.5. Economic consequences of the treatment

It would be paradoxical to devote large sums of money to treatment of hemodialysis patients, and then to refuse these patients any kind of normal activity even when their physical status allows it.

Chronic hemodialysis is today the most expensive of all medical therapy. The French Ministère de la Santé indicates that for 1975 the overall price of one dialysis session is 1168 FF for center dialysis and 556 FF for home dialysis. The annual cost of treatment for three times a week was nearly 150,000 FF in centers and 80,000 FF at home. For all of France, where more than 7,000 patients are treated in 1978, the cost to the national budget reaches approximately 1 billion French Francs per year.

A similar study was conducted by the Artificial Kidney Chronic Uremia Program in 1973 in the U.S.A. Cost per dialysis ranged from 33 to 66 US dollars for the home patient group, 100 to 116 for limited care patients, 144 to 172 for in-center patients and 146 to 259 for home-training units [143]. Among the costs making up these figures, more than 50 percent is for personnel; about 25 percent is for equipment, mainly the use of disposable dialyzers. More recent studies indicate a striking increase in the nation-wide cost of dialysis, exceeding one billion dollars per year in the USA [144]. This is mainly due to the sharp drop in the number of home-treated patients from nearly 40 % in 1972 to about 13 % in 1976 since medicare coverage was extended to treatment of end-stage renal patients in 1972 [145].

These economic considerations do not in any way put in question the value of this treatment. However, they should make the public aware of its high cost and stimulate finding ways of reducing it, while extending the treatment. Three methods of doing this are presently available but insufficiently developed:

— reuse of dialyzers, today practiced in only 20 percent of cases in most European countries;

— development of home dialysis, which not only costs less than in-center dialysis but also provides better clinical result;

— increased renal transplantation with cadever kidneys, which are still in too-short supply in many countries.

In the next years, medical and technological research will no doubt open new ways to palliate renal failure. The extraordinary advances already seen in less than 20 years would seem to bode well for the future.

SUBJECT INDEX

A

Accelerated
  atherosclerosis, 71
Acceptance
  of patients on RDT programs, 11
Accidents
  during dialysis sessions, 52
Acetate ions, in the dialysate, 32
Active
  immunization against virus B, 82
Adequate
  dialysis (criteria), 42
Age
  of patients admitted to RDT, 11
Air
  detector, 29
  embolism, 52
Aliphatic
  amines, 14
Aluminum, 32
  and « dialysis dementia », 77
Amenorrhea, 84
Amicon XM 50®, 35
Ammonia, 14
Androgens, 74
Anemia, 73
Anesthesia
  in the dialysis patient, 85
Angor, 71
  and anemia, 71
  during dialysis sessions, 52
Antibacterial
  agents overdosage, 78
Antihypertensive
  drugs, 58
Anuria, 16
Arterial
  jump grafts, 37
Arteriovenous
  grafts, 37
Arteritis
  of the lower limbs, 71
Ascitis, 84
Atherosclerosis, 71
Autonomous
  system, 76

B

Bacterial
  infections, 81
Basal
  weight, 50
Basic
  principles of dialysis, 19
Bicarbonate ions, 16
Bilatéral
  nephrectomy, 70
Binephrectomy, 70
Blood
  compartment resistance (R), 20
  flow rate, 19, 25
  leak detector, 29
  losses, 73
  pump, 28
Body
  weight, 42
Bone
  biopsy, 78
Bovine
  carotide grafts, 37
Buselmeier
  shunt, 36

C

Calcium
  concentration of the dialysate, 32
  control in dialysis patient, 80
  in city water, 32
Carbohydrate
  metabolism disorders, 82
Cardiac
  arrhythmias (voir hypokalemia), 52
Cardiomyopathy
  (uremic), 73
Cardiovascular
  problems, 70
Cellulose
  acetate, 29
Center dialysis, 40
Cerebrovascular
  accidents, 76
Charcoal
  filters, 33
Chest
  pain, 52
Child, 86

Chills, 52
Chloramines, 32, 73
Cholecalciferol
metabolism disorders, 78
Cholelithiasis, 60
Chromatographic
studies of middle molecules, 15
Cimino-Brescia
fistula, 36
Clearance
(of dialyzers), 27
Clinical
follow-up of RDT, 48
Closed
circuit delivery systems, 29
Coagulation
in the blood circuit, 52
Coil dialyzers, 28
Collapse
(vascular), 60
Comitiality, 54
Compliance, 28
Concentrates
for dialysate fluid, 30
Concentration
gradient, 20
Constipation, 84
Contra-indications
to RDT, 11
Convulsions, 54
Copper, 32, 73
Coronary insufficiency, 58, 71
Counter-current
flow dialysis, 20
Cramps, 54
Creatinine, 13
Creation
of vascular access, 41
Criteria
for initiating RDT, 11
Cumulative
survival rate, 87
Curpophan®, 20
Cylindrical
channels, 24
Cystography, 41

D

Dacron®, 37
Declotting
of vascular access, 39
Deionization, 33

Delivery systems, 29
Demineralization, 33
Depressive
tendency, 78
Diabetic
patients, 86
Dialysance
(of dialyzers), 27
Dialysate
compartment resistance (RD), 20
delivery systems, 29
flow meter, 30
flow rate, 19, 25
fluid composition, 30
Dialysis
encephalopathy (« dialysis dementia »), 77
disequilibrium syndrome, 77
« Dialysis dementia »
(« dialysis encephalopathy »), 77
Dialyzer, 28
permeability coefficient, 20
(principle), 19
Diet
of the dialysis patient, 87
Diffusion
(or conduction transfer), 20
Disorders
of nitrogen metabolism enzymes in uremia, 16
Disposable
dialyzers, 28

E

Early
pericardites, 71
Echocardiography, 72
Economic
consequences of RDT, 89
Effective
dialysis surface area, 20
transmembrane pressure, 23
Elderly
patients, 85
Electrical
breakdown, 54
Electro-encephalogram, 76
Electromagnetic
clamp, 30
Endocarditis (acute), 72
Endocrine
disorders, 84
functions of the kidney, 17
Endogenous
hemolysis, 73
Equipment (hemodialysis), 28

Erythrocyte
  medullary production, 73
Erythropoietin, 17, 73
Evening
  dialysis, 40
Exchange
  transfusion, 56
Excretory
  functions of the kidney, 13

F

Fever, 54
Fibrinolytic
  agents, 39
Fibrous osteitis, 78
First
  hemodialysis sessions, 48
Fistulography, 39
Flow
  rates, 24
Fluid
  intake of the dialysis patient, 88
Fluoride, 32
Fogarty catheter, 39
Formaline, 56
Furosemid, 60

G

Gastralgias, 84
Gastroduodenal
  ulcer, 60
Gastrointestinal
  problems, 84
Glucagon, 82
Glucose
  concentration of the dialysate, 32
Guanidine
  compounds, 13
Guanidinoproprionic
  acid, 14, 73
Guanidinosuccinic
  acid, 14, 74

H

« Hard-water »
  syndrome, 32, 54
Headaches, 56
Heart
  failure, 72
Hematological
  problems, 73
Hematomas, 56

Hemodialysis
  requirements, 12
Hemodynamic
  consequences of fistulae, 39
Hemofiltration, 35
Hemolysis (acute), 56
Hemopericardium, 71
Heparinization, 50
  general heparinization, 50
  regional heparinization, 50
Hepatitis, 60, 81
High-output
  cardiac failure, 39, 72
High-permeability
  membranes, 44
High
  risk dialysis, 11
Histocompatibility
  testing, 41
Hollow-fiber
  dialyzers, 28
Home
  dialysis, 40
Hormonal
  changes in uremia, 15
Hydraulic
  permeability, 23
Hypercalcemia, 54, 56
Hypernatremia, 56
Hypertension, 70
Hypertensive
  episodes during dialysis sessions, 56
Hypertriglyceridemia, 82
Hypocalcemia, 48, 54
Hyponatremia, 56
Hypophyso-gonadal
  axis in uremia, 84
Hypotension
  during dialysis session, 56

I

Immune
  deficiency in uremia, 81
Incidents
  during dialysis sessions, 52
Indications
  for RDT, 11
Individual
  protocol of RDT, 41
Indometacin, 72
Infection
  of vascular access, 37

Infections
  problems, 81
Insulin, 82
Interdialytic
  weight gain, 50
Internal
  fistulas, 36
  resistance of dialyzers to blood flow, 24
Iron, 32
  supplementation, 73

J

« **Jet lesion** », 39

K

Kidney
  diseases leading to chronic renal failure, 11
Kiil « standard »
  dialyzer, 29

L

Laboratory
  follow-up of the dialysis patient, 60
Lasilix, 60
Late pericardites, 72
Left
  ventricular failure, 72
Leukocyte
  alterations, 74
Leukopenia
  during dialysis sessions, 74
Lipid
  metabolism disorders, 82
Limitations
  in dialysis time shortening, 44
Limited-care dialysis, 40
Local
  complications of vascular access, 37
Long-term
  clinical follow-up of RDT, 62
Luteal
  deficiency, 84

M

Manometer
  of blood circuit, 29
  of dialysate circuit, 30
Mass
  solute transfer, 19
Membrane
  resistance (RM), 20
Membranes (dialysis), 19
  rupture, 58

Menorrhage, 58
Mental
  disorders, 78
Metabolic
  functions of the kidney, 17
Metastatic
  calcifications, 80
Methylguanidine, 14, 74
Middle
  molecules, 14
Monitoring
  devices, 29
  of the blood circuit, 29
  of the dialysate fluid, 30
Motor
  nerve-conduction veolocity (MNCV), 76
Multiple-plate
  dialyzers, 28
Multipoint
  parallel-plate dialyzers, 28
Myoinositol, 72
Myocardial
  infarction, 71

N

Neurologic
  complications, 74
  complications related to RDT, 76
Neurological
  accidents of iatrogenic origin, 77
Neuro-muscular
  blocking agents, 85
Nitrates, 32
Nitrites, 32, 73
Nitrogen
  metabolism, 13
Nutritional
  disorders, 82

O

Occlusive
  blood pump, 28
Oligospermia, 84
Organization
  of RDT, 40
Orthostatic
  hypotension, 76
Osteomalacia, 78
Overall
  permeability coefficient, 20
  results of RDT, 87
Overheating
  of dialysate fluid, 56

Overnight
  dialysis, 40
Oxidizing
  filter, 33

P

Pancreatitis, 60
Parallel-plate
  dialyzers, 28
Parathyroidectomy, 81
Parathyroid
  hormon in uremia, 78
Passive
  immunization against virus B, 82
Peptide
  hormones inactivation, 17
Percutaneous
  route, 37
Performance
  (dialyzer), 25
  of dialysis sessions, 48
Pericardial
  friction rub, 71, 72
Pericarditis, 52, 58, 71, 72
Periodic
  laboratory examinations, 62
Phenolic
  compounds, 14, 74
Phosphate
  control in dialysis patient, 80
Phosphocalcic
  metabolism disorders, 78
  product, 80
Platelet
  alterations, 74
  functions in uremia, 74
Poiseuille's laws, 24
Polyacrylonitrite, 20
Polycarbonate, 20
Polycystic
  kidneys
    and anemia, 73
    and infection, 60
Polymethacrylate, 35
Polytetrafluoroethylen, 37
Portable
  conductivity monitor, 56
Potassium
  balance in the dialyzed patient, 16
  concentration of the dialysate, 30
Precordialgias, 58
Predialysis
  levels of nitrogen metabolites, 60
Preparation
  of dialysate concentrates, 32

Pressure drop, 24
Professional
  rehabilitation, 88
Prolonged
  fever, 82
Protamine
  sulfate, 50
Protein
  intake of the dialysis patient, 88
Pruritus, 58, 80
« **Pseudo-gout** », 80
Psychological
  preparation for RDT, 40
Puncture
  point bleeding, 60
Pulmonary
  edema, 58
Pyrogens, 32

Q

Quantitative
  bone histology, 78
Quinton-Scribner
  shunt, 36

R

Rapid
  hemodialysis, 77
Rectangular
  channels, 24
Reducing
  the cost of dialysis, 89
Reduction
  of weekly dialysis time, 44
Redy®
  machine, 29
Renal
  osteodystrophy, 80
  transplantation, 9, 12, 41
Renin-angiotensin
  axis, 17
« **Renin-dependent**
  hypertension, 70
Residual
  diuresis, 42
Resistivimeter, 30
Restless
  legs syndrome, 76
Retrograde
  arterial embolism, 39
Reuse
  of dialyzers, 50
Reverse osmosis, 33
Rhodial®,
  machine, 29

S

Saphenous
    autograft, 37
    homograft, 37

Secondary
    hyperparathyroidism, 78

Sedatives
    overdosage, 78

Sedimentation
    filter, 33

Seizures, 54

Self-care
    dialysis, 40

Semipermeable
    membranes, 19

Sexual
    activity, 84

Sieving
    coefficient (T), 23

Silastic®, 36

Single
    needle dialysis, 50

Sodium
    balance in the dialyzed patient, 16
    concentration of the dialysate, 30, 32
    intake of the dialysis patient, 88

Solvent
    filtration rate (Q_f), 23

Square meter-hour
    hypothesis, 14

Subdural
    hematoma, 77

Sufates, 32

Support
    structures, 28, 29

Surgery
    in the dialysis patient, 85

Surgical
    pericardial drainage, 72

Suspended
    particles, 32

Systemic
    diseases, 85

T

Tachyarrhythmia, 52

Tamponade
    (cardiac), 71

Teflon®, 36

Testosterone
    levels in uremia, 84

Theoretical
    criteria for adequate dialysis, 42

Thermometer, 30

Thomas shunt, 36

Thrombosis
    of vascular access, 37

Thyroid
    hormones in uremia, 84

Trade-off
    hypothesis, 15

Transmittance
    coefficient, 35

Transfer
    (of solutes), 19

Transfusions, 74

Tuberculosis, 81

U

Ultrafiltration
    (or convection transfer), 20
    rate (N), 21
    regulation, 50

Uncontrollable
    hypertension, 70

Urea, 13
    pool, 42

Uremic
    encephalopathy, 76
    polyneurites, 76
    toxicity, 13

Uric
    acid, 13

Urinary
    infection, 81

Vacations, 88

Vascular
    access, 36
    connection, 48

« Vascular steal »
    syndrome, 39

Vitamin
    B_{12} clearance, 42
    D synthetic derivatives, 80
    D_3 metabolism in uremia, 78
    disorders, 82

« Volume-dependent »
    hypertension, 70

Vomiting, 60

W

Water
    and electrolyte excretion, 16
    balance in the dialyzed patient, 16
    softeners, 33
    treatment, 32

Weakness, 73

Weekly
    dialysis time, 42

Weight
    loss during hemodialysis sessions, 50

TABLE OF PLATES

Pl. 1	MAIN KIDNEY DISEASES LEADING TO CHRONIC HEMODIALYSIS	18
Pl. 2	THE STAGES OF CHRONIC RENAL FAILURE	22
Pl. 3	ENDOCRINE FUNCTIONS OF THE KIDNEY	26
Pl. 4	DIFFUSION (OR CONDUCTION) TRANSFER	31
Pl. 5	STRUCTURE OF DIALYSIS MEMBRANES	34
Pl. 6	PRINCIPLES OF ULTRAFILTRATION	38
Pl. 7	PRINCIPAL TYPES OF DIALYZERS	43
Pl. 8	DIALYSATE DELIVERY SYSTEM	46
Pl. 9	CLOSED-CIRCUIT DIALYSIS SYSTEMS	49
Pl. 10	MONITORING DEVICES	51
Pl. 11	WATER TREATEMENT FOR DIALYSIS	53
Pl. 12	HEMOFILTRATION	55
Pl. 13	PERFORMANCE OF DIALYZERS	57
Pl. 14	MAIN TYPES OF VASCULAR ACCESS	59
Pl. 15	HEMODIALYSIS EQUIPMENT	61
Pl. 16	PREPARATION OF DIALYSIS EQUIPMENT	64
Pl. 17	STARTING DIALYSIS SESSION	65
Pl. 18	VASCULAR CONNECTION	66
Pl. 19	HEPARINIZATION AND SURVEILLANCE OF THE DIALYSIS SESSION	67
Pl. 20	END OF DIALYSIS AND BLOOD RESTITUTION	68
Pl. 21	CONTROLS AT THE END OF DIALYSIS	69
Pl. 22	VISCERAL AND METABOLIC DISORDERS OF CHRONIC UREMIA	75
Pl. 23	CALCIUM AND PHOSPHATE DISORDERS	79
Pl. 24	HEPATITIS B : INFECTION IN HEMODIALYSIS CENTERS	83

REFERENCES

1. CROSNIER J. — General concepts of substitute treatment in chronic renal failure. In : *Nephrology,* J. Hamburger, J. Crosnier and J.P. Grunfeld (eds), New York, *John Wiley and Sons,* 1978, in press.
2. SHINABERGER J.H. — Indications for dialysis. In : *Clinical aspects of uremia and dialysis,* S.G. Massry and A.L. Sellers (eds), Springfield, *Charles C. Thomas,* 1976, p. 490.
3. LINDHOLM D.D., BURNELL J.M., MURRAY J.S. — Experience in the treatment of chronic uremia in an outpatient community hemodialysis center. *Trans. Am. Soc. Artif. Intern. Organs.,* **9,** 3, 1963.
4. JUNGERS P., ZINGRAFF J. — Results and limitations of long-term dialysis treatment. In : *Nephrology,* J. Hamburger, J. Crosnier and J.P. Grunfeld (eds), New York, *John Wiley and Sons,* 1978, in press.
5. DEGOULET P., REACH I., AIME S., BERGER C., GOUPY F., JACOBS C., ROJAS P., LEGRAIN M. — Dialysis computer programme. IV. Summary report. The epidemiology of complications. *J. Urol. Nephrol.* (Paris), **83,** 925, 1977.
6. JACOBS C., BRUNNER F.P., CHANTLER C., DONCKERWOLCKE R.A., GURLAND H.J., HATHWAY R.A., SELWOOD N.H., WING A.J. — Combined report on regular dialysis and transplantation in Europe, VII, 1976. *Proc., Eur. Dial. Transpl. Ass.,* **14,** 3, 1977.
7. LOWRIE E.G., LAZARUS J.M., MOCELIN A.J., BAILEY G.L., HAMPERS C.L., XILSON R.E., MERRILL J.P. — Survival of patients undergoing chronic hemodialysis and renal transplantation. *N. Engl. J. Med.,* **288,** 863, 1973.
8. DRUKKER W., HAAGSMA-SCHOUTEN W.A.G., ALBERTS C., SPOEK M.G. — Report on regular dialysis treatment in Europe, V, 1969. *Proc. Eur. Dial. Transpl. Ass.,* **6,** 99, 1969.
9. BOICHIS H., BOTTKANNER G., BARELL V., BARNOACH N., ELIAHOUH H.E. — An epidemiology study of renal failure. I. The need for maintenance hemodialysis. *Am. J. Epidem.,* **101,** 276, 1975.
10. JUNGERS P., MANN N.K. — Uremic toxicity. In : *Nephrology.* J. Hamburger, J. Crosnier and J.P. Grunfeld (eds), New York, *John Wiley and Sons,* 1978, in press.
11. JOHNSON W.J., HAGGE W.W., WAGONER R.D., DINAPOLI R.P., ROSEVEAR J.W. — Toxicity arising from urea. *Kidney Int.,* **7,** S 288, 1975.
12. JONES J.D., BURNETT P.C. — Creatinine metabolism and toxicity. *Kidney Int.,* **7,** S 294, 1975.
13. HOROWITZ H.I., STEIN I.M., COHEN B.D., WHITE J.G. — Further studies on the platelet inhibitory effect of guanidinosuccinic acid and its role in uremia bleeding. *Am. J. Med.,* **49,** 336, 1970.
14. SCHREINER G.E., MAHER J.F. — Uremia and the gastro-intestinal tract. In : *Uremia : biochemistry, pathogenesis and treatment.* Springfield Charles C. Thomas, 1971, p. 331.
15. SCRIBNER B.H., BABB A.L. — Evidence for toxins of « middle » molecular weight. *Kidney Int.,* **7,** S 349, 1975.
16. BABB A.L., POPOVICH R.P., CHRISTOPHER T.G., SCRIBNER B.H. — The genesis of the square meter-hour hypothesis. *Trans. Am. Soc. Artif. Intern. Organs.,* **17,** 81, 1971.
17. FUNCK-BRENTANO J.L., MAN N.K., SAUSSE A., CUEILLE G., ZINGRAFF J., DRUEKE T., JUNGERS P., BILLON J.P. — Neuropathy and « middle » molecules toxins. *Kidney Int.,* **7,** S 352, 1975.
18. BERGSTROM J., FURST P. — Uremic middle molecules. *Clin. Nephrol.,* **5,** 143, 1976.
19. MAN N.K., CUEILLE G., ZINGRAFF J., DRUEKE T., JUNGERS P., BILLON J.P., SAUSSE A., FUNCK-BRENTANO J.L. — Investigations on clinico-chemical correlations in uraemic polyneuritis. *Proc. Eur. Dial. Transpl. Ass.,* **11,** 214, 1974.
20. BRICKER N.S. — On the pathogenesis of the uremic state : an exposition of the « trade-off hypothesis ». *N. Engl. J. Med.,* **286,** 1093, 1972.
21. JUNGERS P. — Nitrogen retention. In : *Nephrology.* J. Hamburger, J. Crosnier and J.P. Grunfeld (eds), New York, *John Wiley and Sons,* 1978, in press.
22. GRUNFELD J.P. — Analytical study of renal excretion of water and electrolytes in chronic renal failure. In : *Nephrology,* J. Hamburger, J. Crosnier and J.P. Grunfeld (eds), New York, *John Wiley and Sons,* 1978, in press.
23. MULROW P.J. — Renal hormones. In : *The Kidney,* B.M. Brenner and F.C. Rector (eds), Philadelphia, *W.B. Saunders,* 1976, p. 477-492.

24. DE LUCA H.F. — The kidney as an endocrine organ involved in the function of vitamin D. *Am. J. Med.*, **58**, 39, 1975.

25. MAN N.K., JUNGERS P. — Basic principles of dialysis. In : *Nephrology*, J. Hamburger, J. Crosnier and J.P. Grunfeld (eds), New York, *John Wiley and Sons*, 1978, in press.

26. WOLF A.V., REMP D.G., KILEY J.E., CURRIE G.D. — Artificial kidney function : kinetics of hemodialysis. *J. Clin. Invest.*, **30**, 1062, 1951.

27. MICHAELS A.S. — Operating parameters and performance criteria for hemodialyzers and other membrane-separation devices. *Trans. Am. Soc. Artif. Intern. Organs.*, **17**, 81, 1971.

28. HAMPERS C.L., SCHUPAK E., LOWRIE E.G., LAZARUS J.M. — Clinical engineering in hemodialysis. In : *Long-term hemodialysis*, 2d edition New York, *Grune and Stratton*, 1973, p. 32.

29. LEONARD E.F., BLUEMLE L.W. Jr. — The permeability concept as applied to dialysis. *Trans. Am. Soc. Artif. Intern. Organs.*, **6**, 33, 1960.

30. GREEN D.M., ANTWILER G.D., MONCRIEF, J.W. DECHERD J.F., POPOVICH R.P. — Measurement of the transmittance coefficient-spectrum of Cuprophan and RP 6 membranes : application to the middle molecule removal via ultrafiltration. *Trans. Am. Soc. Artif. Int. Organs.*, **22**, 627, 1976.

31. MAN N.K., GRANGER A., RONDON-NUCETE M., ZINGRAFF J., JUNGERS P., SAUSSE A., FUNCK BRENTANO J.L. — One year follow up of short dialysis with a membrane highly permeable to middle molecules. *Proc. Eur. Dial. Transpl. Ass.*, **10**, 236, 1973.

32. GOTCH F.A. — Solute transport and ultra-filtration in hemodialysis. In : *Clinical aspects of uremia and dialysis*, S.G. Massry and A.L. Sellers (eds), Springfield, *Charles C. Thomas*, 1976, p. 639.

33. KOLFF W.J. WATSCHINGER B. — Further development of a Coil Kindney. Disposable artificial kidney. *J. Lab. Clin. Med.*, **47**, 969, 1956.

34. LOWRIE E.G., HAMPERS C.L., MERRILL J.P. — Twin coil : performance and predictability. *Trans. Am. Soc. Artif. Intern. Organs.*, **15**, 60, 1969.

35. KIIL F. — Development of a parallel flow artificial kidney in plastics. *Acta. chir. scand.*, **253**, S 143, 1960.

36. EDSON H.B., KEEN M.L., GOTCH F.A. — Comparative solute transport and therapeutic effectiveness of multiple point support and standard Kiil hemodialyzers. *Trans. Am. Soc. Artif. intern. Organs.*, **18**, 113, 1972.

37. KERR D.N.S., HOENICH N.A., FROST T.H. — Progress in hemodialysis 1974-1975. In : *Advances in Nephrology*, **6**, 415, 1976.

38. GOTCH F., SARGENT, KEEN M., HOLMES G., TEISINGER C. — Development of long term clinical evaluation of a thrombo-resistant hollow fiber kidney (HFK). *Trans. Am. Soc. Artif. intern. Organs*, **18**, 135, 1972.

39. GORDON A., BETTER O.S., GREENBAUM M.A., MARANTZ L.B., GRAL T., MAXWELL M.H. — Clinical maintenance hemodialysis with a sorbent-based, low-volume dialysate regeneration system. *Trans. Am. Soc. Artif. intern. Organs.*, **17**, 253, 1971.

40. DRUEKE T., BORDIER P.J., MAN N.K., JUNGERS P., MARIE P. — Effects of high dialysate calcium concentration on bone remodelling, serum biochemistry and parathyroid hormone in patients with renal osteodystrophy. *Kidney Int.*, **11**, 267, 1977.

41. JOHNSON G.J. — Optimum dialysate calcium concentration during maintenance hemodialysis. *Nephron*, **17**, 241, 1976.

42. MION C.M., HEGSTROM R.M., BOENS T., SCRIBNER B.H. — Substitution of sodium acetate for sodium bicarbonate in the bath fluid for hemodialysis. *Trans. Am. Soc. Artif. Intern. Organs.*, **10**, 110, 1964.

43. COMTY C., LUEHMANN D., WATHEN R., SHAPIRO F. — Prescription water for chronic hemodialysis. *Trans. Am. Soc. Artif. Intern. Organs.* **20**, 189, 1974.

44. FREEMAN R.M., LAWTON R.L., CHAMBERLAIN M.A. — Hard-water syndrome. *N. Engl. J. Med.*, **276**, 1113, 1967.

45. ALFREY A.C., LEGENDRE G.R., KAEHNY W.D. — The dialysis encephalopathy syndrome. Possible aluminum intoxication. *N. Engl. J. Med.*, **294**, 184, 1976.

46. MADSEN R.F., NIELSEN B., OLSEN O.J., RAASCHOU F. — Reverse osmosis as a method of preparing dialysis water. *Nephron*, **7**, 545, 1970.

47. HENDERSON L.W., BESARAB A., MICHALES A., BLUEMLE L.W. — Blood purification by ultrafiltration and fluid replacement (diafiltration). *Trans. Am. Soc. Artif. Intern. Organs.*, **13**, 216, 1967.

48. COLTON C.K., HENDERSON L.W., FORD C.A., LYSAGHT M.J. — Kinetics of hemodiafiltration. I. In vitro transport characteristics of a hollow-fiber bood ultrafilter. *J. Lab. Clin. Med.*, **85**, 355, 1975.

49. QUELLHORST A., RIEGER J., GOHT B., BECKMANN H., JACOB I., KRAFT B., MIETZSCH G., SCHELER F. — Treatment of chronic uraemia by an ultrafiltration kidney. First clinical experience. *Proc., Eur. Dial. Transpl. Ass.* **13,** 314, 1976.

50. MAN N.K., FUNCK-BRENTANO J.L. — Hemofiltration, an alternative method for treatment of end-stage renal failure. *Advances in Nephrology,* **7,** 293, 1977.

51. JUNGERS P., MAN N.K. — Organization of chronic dialysis and patient follow-up in *Nephrology,* Hamburger J., Crosnier J., and Grunfeld J.P. (eds), New York, *John Wiley and Sons,* 1978, in press.

52. BARBOUR B.H., BERNSTEIN M., CANTOR P.A., FISHER B.S., STONE W. Jr — Clinical use of NSR 440 polycarbonate membrane for hemodialysis, *Trans. Am. Soc. Artif. Intern. Organs.,* **21,** 144, 1975.

53. SCRIBNER B.J., CANER J.E.Z., BURI R., QUINTON W. — The technique of continuous hemodialysis. *Trans. Am. Soc. Artif. Intern. Organs.,* **6,** 88, 1960.

54. BRESCIA M.J., CIMINO J.E., APPEL K., HURWITH B.J. — Chronic hemodialysis using venipuncture and a surgically created arteriovenous fistula. *N. Engl. J. Med.,* **275,** 1089, 1966.

55. BUTT K.M.H., KOUNTZ S.L., FRIEDMAN E.A. — Angioaccess for hemodialysis : which, when, why. *Clin. Nephrol.,* **3,** 207, 1975.

56. QUINTON W.E., DILLARD D.H., SCRIBNER B.H. — Cannulation of blood vessels for prolonged hemodialysis. *Trans. Am. Soc. Artif. Intern. Organs.,* **6,** 104, 1960.

57. BUSELMEIER T.J., SIMMONS R.L., NAJARIAN J.S., DUNCAN D.A. VON HARTITSCH B., KJELLSTRAND C.M. — The clinical application of a new prosthetic arteriovenous shunt, *Nephron,* **12,** 22, 1973.

58. THOMAS G.I. — A large vessel applique arteriovenous shunt for dialysis. *Trans. Am. Soc. Artif. Intern. Organs.,* **15,** 288, 1969.

59. JOHNSON J.M., KENOYER M.R., JOHNSON K.E., POTTER D.J., NICKAS G.M., WILLIAMS T. — The modified bovine heterograft in vascular access for chronic hemodialysis. *Ann. Surgery,* **183,** 62, 1976.

60. BAKER L.D., JOHNSON J.M., GOLDFARB D. — Expanded polytetrafluorethylene (P.T.F.E.) subcutaneous arteriovenous conduit : an improved vascular access for chronic hemodialysis. *Trans. Am. Soc. Artif. Intern. Organs.,* **22,** 382, 1976.

61. HAIMOV H., BAEZ A., NEFF M., SLIFKIN R. — Complications of arteriovenous fistulas for hemodialysis. *Arch. Surgery,* **110,** 708, 1975.

62. GAAN D., MALLICK N.P., BREWIS R.A.L., SEEDAT Y.K. — Cerebral damage from declotting Scribner shunts. *Lancet,* **2,** 77, 1969.

63. ANDERSON C.B., CODD J.P., GRAFF R.A., GROCE M.A., HARTER H.R., NEWTON W.T. — Cardiac failure and upper extremity arteriovenous dialysis fistulas. *Arch. Intern. Med.,* **136,** 292, 1976.

64. BLAGG C.R., HICKMAN R.O., ESCHBACH J.W., SCRIBNER B.H. — Home hemodialysis : six years experience. *N. Engl. J. Med.,* **283,** 1126, 1970.

65. BAILLOD R.A., COMTY C., ILAHI M., KONOTEY-AHULU F.I.D., SEVITT L., SHALDON S. — Overnight haemodialysis in the home. *Proc., Eur. Dial. Transpl. Assoc.,* **2,** 99, 1965.

66. ROBERTS J.L. — Analysis and outcome of 1063 patients trained for home hemodialysis. *Kidney Int.,* **9,** 363, 1976.

67. SIEMSEN A.W., ENNIS J., Mc GOWAN R., WONG E.G.C., WONG L.M.F. — Limited-care hemodialysis — *Trans. Am. Soc. Artif. Intern. Organs.,* **18,** 70, 1972.

68. MARTIN A.M., ODURO-DOMINAH A., GIBBINS J.K., DEVAPAL D., MITCHELL D.C. — Regular short haemodialysis in end-stage renal failure, *Br. Med., J.,* **3,** 758, 1975.

69. DE PALMA J.R., ABUKURAH A., RUBINI M.E. — Adequacy of hemodialysis. *Proc. Eur. Dial. Transpl. Assoc.,* **9,** 265, 1972.

70. BARBER S., APPLETON D.R., KERR D.N.S. — Adequate dialysis. *Nephron,* **14,** 209, 1975.

71. BABB A.L., FARRELL P.C., UVELLI D.A., SCRIBNER B.H. — Hemodialyzer evaluation by examination of solute molecular spectra. *Trans. Am. Soc. Artif. Intern. Organs.,* **18,** 98, 1972.

72. BABB A.L., STRAND M.J., UVELLI D.A., MILUTINOVIC J., SCRIBNER B.H. — Quantitative description of dialysis treatment : a dialysis index. *Kidney Int.,* **7,** S 23, 1975.

73. SARGENT J.A., GOTCH F.A. — The analysis of concentration dependence of uremic lesions in clinical studies. *Kidney Int.,* **7,** S 35, 1975.

74. PETERS J.H., GOTCH F.A., KEEN M., BERRIDGE B.J. Jr.,CHAO W.R. — Investigation of the clearance and generation rate of endogenous peptides in normal subjects and uremic patients. *Trans. Am. Soc. Artif. Intern. Organs.,* **20,** 417, 1974.

75. MILUTINOVIC J., STRAND M., CASARETTO A., FOLETTE W., BABB A., SCRIBNER B.H. — Clinical impact of residual glomerular filtration rate on dialysis time : a preliminary report. *Trans. Am. Soc. Artif. Intern. Organs.,* **20**, 410, 1974.
76. GOTCH F.A., SARGENT J.A., KEEN M., LAM M., PROWITT M., GRADY M. — Clinical results of intermittent dialysis therapy guided by ongoing kinetic analysis of urea metabolism. *Trans. Am. Soc. Artif. Intern. Organs.,* **22**, 175, 1976.
77. ARIEFF A.I., MASSRY S.G., BARRIENTOS A., KLEEMAN C.R., — Brain water and electrolyte metabolism in uremia : effects of slow and rapid hemodialysis. *Kidney Int.,* **4**, 177, 1973.
78. POPOVICH R.P., HLAVINKA D.J., BOMAR J.B., MONCRIEF J.W., DECHERD J.F. — The consequences of physiological resistances of metabolic removal from the patient artificial kidney system. *Trans. Am. Soc. Artif. Intern. Organs.,* **21**, 108, 1975.
79. ZINGRAFF J., RONDON NUCETE M., DRUEKE T., ROUX J.P., MAN N.K., JUNGERS P. — Bilateral fracture of the femoral neck complicating uremic bone disease prior to chronic hemodialysis. *Clin. Nephrol.,* **3**, 73, 1974.
80. KOPP K.F., VOGEL G., SCHMIDT U., PISTER H., HUGHES S., VAN DURA D., RAMIREZ G., GUTCH C.F., KOLFF W.J. — An up-to-date appraisal of single needle dialysis, *Proc. Eur. Dial. Transpl. Ass.,* **11**, 167, 1974.
81. WARD M.K., SHADFORTH M., HILL A.V.L., KERR D.N.S. — Air embolism during hemodialysis. *Br. Med. J.,* **3**, 1971.
82. NICKEY W.A., CHINITZ V.L., KIM K.E., ONESTI G., SWARTZ C. — Hypernatremia from water softener malfunction during home dialysis. *J. Am. Med. Ass.,* **214**, 915, 1970.
83. FORTNER R.W., NOWAKOWSKI A., CARTER C.B., KING L.H., KNEPSHIELD J.H. — Death due to overheated dialysate during dialysis. *Ann. Intern. Med.,* **73**, 443, 1970.
84. ORRINGER E.P., MATTERN W.D. — Formaldehyde-induced hemolysis during chronic hemodialysis. *N. Engl. J. Med.,* **294**, 1416, 1976.
85. WEIDMANN P., MAXWELL M.H. — Hypertension, in : *Clinical Aspects of Uremia and Dialysis,* S.G. Massry and A.C. Sellers (eds), Springfield, *Charles C. Thomas,* 1976, p. 100.
86. DESCHAMPS A., GRUNFELD J.P., ZINGRAFF J., DRUEKE T., JUNGERS P. — Hypertension artérielle et mortalité par accident cardio-vasculaire chez les hémodialysés chroniques. *Arch. Mal. Cœur* (Paris), 1978, sous presse.
87. SAFAR M., LONDON G.M., WEISS Y.A., MILLIEZ P.L. — Overhydration and renin in hypertensive patients with terminal renal failure : a hemodynamic study. *Clin. Nephrol.,* **5**, 183, 1975.
88. BAGDADE J.D. — Atherosclerosis in patients undergoing maintenance hemodialysis. *Kidney Int.,* **7**, S 370, 1975.
89. LINDNER A., CHARRA B., SHERRARD D.J., SCRIBNER B.H. — Accelerated atherosclerosis in prolonged maintenance hemodialysis. *N. Engl. J. Med.,* **290**, 697, 1974.
90. BAGDADE J.D., PORTE D.Jr., BIERMAN E.L. — Hypertriglyceridemia : a metabolic consequence of renal failure. *N. Engl. J. Med.,* **279**, 181, 1968.
91. CATTRAN D.C., STEINER G., FENTON S.S.A., WILSON D.R. — Hypertriglyceridemia in uremia and the use of triglyceride turnover to define pathogenesis. *Trans. Am. Soc. Artif. Intern. Organs.,* **20**, 148, 1974.
92. LAZARUS J.M., LOWRIE, E.G., HAMPERS C.L., MERRILL J.P. — Cardiovascular disease in uremic patients on hemodialysis. *Kidney Int.,* **7**, S 167, 1975.
93. MARINI P.V., HULL A.R. — Uremic pericarditis : a review of incidence and management. *Kidney int.,* **7**, S 163, 1975.
94. JUNGERS P., ZINGRAFF J., MAN N.K., DRUEKE T., CROSNIER J. — Uremic pericarditis : experience in 1007 chronic hemodialysis patients (in preparation).
95. COMTY C.M., COHEN S.I., SHAPIRO F.L. — Pericarditis in chronic uremia and its sequels. *Ann. Intern. Med.,* **75**, 173, 1971.
96. CROSS A.S., STEIGBIGEL R.T. — Infective endocarditis and access site infections in patients on hemodialysis, *Medicine,* **55**, 6, 1976.
97. DRUEKE T., LE PAILLEUR C., MEILHAC B., KOUTOUDIS C., ZINGRAFF J., DI MATTEO J., CROSNIER J. — Congestive cardiomyopathy in uraemic patients. *Br. Med. J.,* **1**, 350, 1977.
98. BREZIN J.H., LYONS P. — Cardiomyopathy in uraemic patients on long term haemodialysis. *Br. Med. J.,* **1**, 976, 1977.

99. ESCHBACH J.W., HARKER L.A., DALE D.C. — The hematological consequences of renal failure, in : *The Kidney,* by M. Brenner et E. Rector, Philadelphia, *W.B. Saunders* 1976, 2 vol., p. 1522.

100. ESCHBACH J.W. Jr, FUNK D., ADAMSON J., KUHN I., SCRIBNER B.H., FINCH C.A. — Erythropoiesis in patients with renal failure undergoing chronic dialysis. *N. Engl. J. Med.,* **276,** 653, 1967.

101. ZINGRAFF J., DRUEKE T., MARIE P., MAN N.K., JUNGERS P., BORDIER Ph. — Anemia and secondary hyperparathyroidism. *Arch. Int. Med.,* 1978 (in press).

102. BARSOTTI G., BEVILACQUA G., MORELLI E., CAPPELLI P., BALESTRI P.L., GIOVANNETTI S. — Toxicity arising from guanidine compounds : role of methylguanidine as a uremic toxin. *Kidney Int.,* **7,** S 299, 1975.

103. SHAINKIN R., GIATT Y., BERLYNE G.M. — The presence and toxicity of guanidino proprionic acid in uremia. *Kidney Int.,* **7,** S 302, 1975.

104. HENDLER E.D., GOFFINET J.A., ROSS S., LONGNECKER R.E., BAROVIC V. — Controlled study of androgen therapy in anemia of patients on maintenance hemodialysis. *N. Engl. J. Med.,* **291,** 1046, 1975.

105. BRUBAKER L.H., JENSEN D., JOHNSON C., NORTHUM R., NOLPH K.D. — Kinetics of stagnation-induced neutropenia during hemodialysis. *Trans. Am. Soc. Artif. Intern. Organs.,* **18,** 305, 1972.

106. CRADDOCK P.R., FEHR J., DALMASSO A.P., BRIGHAM K.L., JACOB H.S. — Hemodialysis leukopenia. Pulmonary vascular leukostasis resulting from complement activation by dialyzer cellophane membranes. *J. Clin. Invest.,* **59,** 879, 1977.

107. EKNOYAN G., WACKSMAN S.J., GLUECK H.I., WILL J.J. — Platelet function in renal failure. *N. Engl. J. Med.,* **280,** 677, 1969.

108. HOROWITZ H.I., STEIN I.M., COHEN B.D., WHITE J.G. — Further studies on the platelet-inhibitory effect of guanidinosuccinic acid and its role in uremia bleeding. *Am. J. Med.,* **49,** 336, 1970.

109. RABINER S.F., MOLINAS F. — The role of phenol and phenolic acids on the thrombocytopathy and defective platelet aggregation of patients with renal failure. *Am. J. Med.,* **49,** 346, 1970.

110. RASKIN N.H., FISHMAN R.A. — Neurologic disorders in renal failure. *N. Engl. J. Med.,* **294,** 204, 1976.

111. TESCHAN P.E., GINN H.E., WALKER P.J., BOURNE J.R., FRISTOE M., WARD J.W. — Quantified functions of the nervous system in uremic patients on maintenance dialysis. *Trans. Am. Soc. Artif. Intern. Organs.,* **20,** 388, 1974.

112. DYCK P.J., JOHNSON W.J., LAMBERT E.H., BUSHEK W., POLLOCK M. — Detection and evaluation of uremic peripheral neuropathy in patients on hemodialysis. *Kidney Int.,* **7,** S 201, 1975.

113. TYLER H.R. — Uremic neuritis and the autonomic system. *N. Engl. J. Med.,* **290,** 685, 1974.

114. NIELSEN V.K. — The peripheral nerve function in chronic renal failure. VII : longitudinal course during terminal renal failure and regular hemodialysis. *Acta. Med. Scand.,* **195,** 155, 1974.

115. NIELSEN V.K. — The peripheral nerve function in chronic renal failure. IV. An analysis of vibratory perception threshold. *Acta. Med. Scand.,* **191,** 287, 1972.

116. LEONARD C.D., WEIL E., SCRIBNER B.H. — Subdural hematomas in patients undergoing hemodialysis. *Lancet,* **2,** 239, 1969.

117. ARIEFF A.I., MASSRY S.G. — Dialysis disequilibrium syndrome, in : *Clinical aspects of uremia and dialysis.* S.G. Massry and A.L. Sellers (eds), Springfield, *Charles C. Thomas,* 1976, p. 34.

118. ALFREY A.C., MISHELL J.M., BURKS J., CONTIGUGLIA S.R., RUDOLPH H., LEWIN E., HOLMES J.H. — Syndrome of dyspraxia and multifocal seizures associated with chronic hemodialysis. *Trans. Am. Soc. Artif. Intern. Organs.,* **18,** 257, 1972.

119. KAENHY W.D., ALFREY A.E., HOLMAN R.E., SHORR W.J. — Aluminum transfer during hemodialysis. *Kidney Int.,* **12,** 361, 1977.

120. BENNETT W.M., SINGER I., GOLPER T., FEIG P., COGGINS C.J. — Guidelines for drug therapy in renal failure. *Ann. Intern. Med.,* **86,** 754, 1977.

121. MASSRY S.G., COBURN J.W. — Divalent ion metabolism and renal osteodystrophy, in : *Clinical Aspects of Uremia and Dialysis.* Massry S.G. and Sellers A.L. eds, Springfield, *Charles C. Thomas* 1976 p. 304-387.

122. BORDIER Ph., ZINGRAFF J., DRUEKE T. — Renal osteodystrophy, in : *Nephrology,* Hamburger J., Crosnier J. and Grunfeld J.P. (eds), New York, *John Wiley and Sons,* 1978, in presse.

123. FOURNIER A.E., ARNAUD C.D., JOHNSON W.J., TAYLOR W.F., GOLDSMITH R.S. — Etiology of hyperparathyroïdism and bone disease during chronic hemodialysis. II. Factors affecting serum immunoreactive parathyroid hormone. *J. Clin. Invest.,* **50,** 126, 1971.

124. HRUSKA K.A., KOPELMAN R., RUTHERFORD W.E., KLAHR S., SLATOPOLSKY E. —

Metabolism of immunoreactive parathyroid hormone in the dog. The role of the kidney and the effects of chronic renal disease. *J. Clin. Invest.,* **56,** 39, 1975.

125. BRICKMAN A.S., COBURN J.W., FRIEDMAN G.R., OKAMURA W.H., MASSRY S.G., NORMAN A.W. — Comparison of effects of 1 alpha hydroxy vitamin D and 1,25 dihydroxy vitamine D 3. *J. Clin. Invest.,* **57,** 1540, 1976.

126. BORDIER Ph., ZINGRAFF J., GUERIS J., JUNGERS P., MARIE P., PECHET M., RASMUSSEN H. — The effect of 1 alpha (OH) D3 and 1 alpha, 25 (OH) D3 on the bone in patients with renal osteodystrophy. *Am. J. Med.,* **64,** 101, 1978.

127. EASTWOOD J.B., BORDIER Ph., CLARKSON E.M., TUN CHOT S., de WARDENER H.E. — The contrasting effects on bone histology of vitamin D and of calcium carbonate in the osteomalacia of chronic renal failure. *Clin. Sci.,* **47,** 23, 1974.

128. DOBBELSTEIN H., KORNER W.F., MEMPEL W., GROSSZ-WILDE H., EDEL H.H. — Vitamin B6 deficiency in uremia and its implications for the depression of immune responses. *Kidney Int.,* **5,** 233, 1974.

129. SOULIER J.P., JUNGERS P., ZINGRAFF J. — Virus B hepatitis in hemodialysis centers. *Advances in Nephrology,* **6,** 383, 1976.

130. BLUMBERG B.S., SUTNIK A.J., LONDON W.T. — Australia Antigen as a hepatitis virus. Variation in host response. *Am. J. Med.,* **48,** 1, 1970.

131. LONDON W.T., DREW J.S., LUSTBADER E.D., WERNER B.G., BLUMBERG B.S. — Host responses to hepatitis B infection in patients in a chronic hemodialysis unit. *Kidney Int.,* **12,** 51, 1977.

132. Public Health Laboratory Service Survey. Hepatitis B in retreat from dialysis units in United Kingdom. *Br. Med., J.,* **1,** 1579, 1976.

133. DELONS S., NARET C., CIANCIONI C., COUROUCE A.M., SOULIER J.P. — An attempt to prevent B-hepatitis in a hemodialysis unit's team. Utilization of specific immunoglobulins. *Proc. Eur. Dial. Transpl. Ass.,* **11,** 237, 1974.

134. BAGDADE J.D. — Disorders of glucose metabolism in uremia. *Advances in Nephrology,* **8,** 1978, in press.

135. SANFELIPO M.L., SWENSON R.S., REAVEN G.M. — Reduction of plasma triglycerides by diet in subjects with chronic renal failure. *Kidney Int.,* **11,** 54, 1977.

136. KOPPLE J.D., SWENDSEID M.E., SHINABERGER J.H., UMEZAWA C.Y. — The free and bound amino-acids removed by hemodialysis. *Trans. Am. Soc. Artif. Intern. Organs,* **14,** 309, 1973.

137. LIM V.S., FANG V.S. — Gonadal dysfunction in uremic men. A study of hypothalamio-pituitary-testicular axis before and after renal transplantation. *Am. J. Med.,* **58,** 655, 1975.

138. ZINGRAFF J., JUNGERS P., PELISSIER C., FEINSTEIN M.C., ROGER M., SCHOLLER R. — Hormonal study of hypothalamie-pituitary-ovarian axls in uremic women (in preparation).

139. BAILEY G.L., MOCELIN A.J., GRIFFITHS J.J.L., ZSCHAECK D., GHANTOUS W.N., HAMPERS C.L., MERRILL J.P., WILSON R.E. — Hemodialysis and renal transplantation in patients of the 50-80 age group. *J. Am. Geriatr. Soc.,* **20,** 421, 1972.

140. SHAPIRO F.L., KJELLSTRAND C.M., GOETZ F.C. — End-stage diabetic nephropathy, *Kidney Int.,* **6,** 1, S 1-186, 1974.

141. BROYER M. — Treatment of chronic renal failure in children, *in : Nephrology,* Hamburger J., Crosnier J. and Grunfeld J.P. (eds), New York, *John Wiley and Sons,* 1978, in press.

142. CHANTLER C., DONCKERWOLCKE R.A., BRUNNER F.P., GURLAND H.J., HATHWAY R.A., JACOBS C., SELWOOD N.H., WING A.J. — Combined report on regular dialysis and transplantation of children in Europe, 1976, *Proc. Eur. Dial. Transpl. Ass.,* **14,** 70, 1977.

143. HOFFSTEIN P.A., KRUEGER K.K., WINEMAN R.J. — Dialysis costs : results of a diverse sample study. *Kidney Int.,* **9,** 286, 1976.

144. STANGE P.V., SUMMER A.T. — Predicting treatment costs and life expectancy for endstage renal disease. *N. Engl. J. Med.,* **298,** 372, 1978.

145. FRIEDMAN E.A., DELANO B.G., BUTT K.M.H. — Pragmatic realities in uremia therapy. *N. Engl. J. Med.,* **298,** 368, 1978.